Learn Yourself

VEDIC ASTROLOGY

IN 15 DAYS

By

B. Suryanarain Rao

SURA BOOKS (Pvt) LTD.
(An ISO 9000 Certified Company)
Chennai • Ernakulam

Price: Rs.80.00

LEARN YOURSELF VEDIC ASTROLOGY IN 15 DAYS

BY

B. Suryanarain Rao

First Edition : June, 2006

Size : ⅛ Demy

Pages : 208

Price: Rs.80.00

ISBN: 81-7478-830-1

SURA BOOKS (PVT) LTD.

Head Office:
1620, 'J' Block,
16th Main Road,
Anna Nagar,
Chennai - 600040.
Phones: 26162173, 26161099.

Branch:
XXXII/2328, New Kalavath Road,
Opp. to BSNL, Near Chennoth Glass,
Palarivattom,
Ernakulam - 682025.
Phone: 0484-3205797.

Printed at T. Krishna Press, Chennai - 600 102 and
Published by V.V.K.Subburaj for Sura Books (Pvt) Ltd.,
1620, 'J' Block, 16th Main Road, Anna Nagar, Chennai - 600 040.
Phones: 26162173, 26161099. Fax: (91) 44-26162173.
email: surabooks@eth.net; website: www.surabooks.com

CONTENTS

Page

SCIENTIFIC INTRODUCTION

I was the first to write on Astrology in English in India. A small book under the title "A Short Compendium of Astrology" published in 1882 and another work called the "Astrological Self-Instructor" in 1892, sold rapidly. This encouraged me to simplify and publish such pamphlets as this would easily enable the ordinary public, to cast their own horoscopes and to know the principal events of their lives—past, present and future. The books are addressed to the semi-scientific readers and these form the overwhelming majority of the educated public. The advanced student of the Astrological science will find a little which he does not already know, and those who are utterly ignorant of the first elements of science, will be able to understand or feel an interest in formulas which have been explained in the following pages. The general object kept in view in writing this book has been to produce something from which a student might derive a clear, comprehensive and distinct knowledge of Astrology.

A few facts given here for the information of the readers will clearly and scientifically show that men are under the direct influence of the planets – physically, mentally and financially.

Each Animal gets Sun's Energy and Power

I shall work one or two figures to show what minute fraction of the Sun's energy is sufficient to call a man into existence and destroy him again. Let it be supposed for one moment that the Earth contains only men and their number is fixed roughly at 2,000 millions. Each man then wants $\frac{1}{4,000,000,000,000,000,000}$ part of the Solar power radiated into space. Consider again for a moment that the earth is composed only of animals and think there are one billion of them. Then each animal gets

$\frac{1}{2,000,000,000,000,000,000,000}$ th energy. Of course, these are absurd guesses. The Earth is composed of so many millions, billions, trillions etc. of animals, vegetables and minerals that no adequate idea can be formed of its hugeness or the inconceivable fraction of the Solar power required to call the individual bodies into existence. The confusion of mathematical figure will be hopeless and unsolvable. A drop of blood of the musk deer held by the point of a fine needle contains millions of living corpuscles or organisms. Gravitation is exerted in various degrees by every mass of matter upon every other mass in the Universe. The Sun is a huge mass of matter and its gravitation must be on a corresponding magnitude. There are more than 180 planets, but most of them are insignificant and do not exercise any perceptible influence upon the earthly phenomena.

Sun is the Chief planet

Seven planets have been marked by the significant names by the ancients. Everything on the surface of the Earth is subjected to terrestrial gravity, but the other components of the Universe also exercise their attraction upon us. It has been demonstrated, that the most important planets reflect the solar energy greatly modified and their influences upon terrestrial phenomena have been ascertained. Without the solar influence there could neither be rain, nor springs, nor rivers nor oceans. Rains are dependent upon currents in the atmosphere and these are distributed by Solar heat and the electrical currents which accompany heat rays. The manifestation of vegetable or animal life is entirely due to solar light and heat. In fact, the great changes experienced at different epochs of the world's history, whether natural, political, social, religious or intellectual are entirely due to our varying relations with the Sun, with whom everyone of us is familiar, but about whose tremendous influence on the globe, the greater we try to know, the greater remains for us to know. Water is converted into vapour by the solar rays; vapour rises into the atmosphere, is condensed, there, by cold blasts of winds, falls down as rain and dew, supports vegetation and nourishes animal and man. Man is the creature of circumstances and readily adapts himself to them. Morning Sun is bilious, while evening Sun is healthy and the change is demonstrable. Fine mornings exhilarate men and gloomy mornings depress their spirits. The Sun's rays when refracted, undergo remarkable changes, and the seven colours into which they are refracted viz. violet, indigo, blue, green, yellow, orange and red, exhibit marked heating effects and the slightest irregularities in surface, are enough to produce unperceived refractions and the consequent changes in the chemical effects. No man can say that he does not influence nature or Nature does not influence him.

Climatic Effects due to Solar Rays

Heat and cold, wind and rain, magnetism and the earlier stages of the planetary revolutions, the wonderful endless variety of phenomena is due to thousands of causes which have been at work under the all-controlling power of the solar rays. By carefully studying this, it is possible to predict their character, existence, development and final destruction. These are not the results of blind chance, working without any purpose. The Sun's rays determine the climate of a place. Herschell observes "The principal factor in the formation of climate is of course solar heat, the climate of any place is depending primarily on the lengths of the days and nights and on the relative duration of the sessions. But climate is also greatly affected by the nature of the surface, whether it be land or water. Water parts with its heat more slowly than the land does, and it thus retains a store, which serves to equalize the temperature. On land again, the climate depends to a very great extent on the altitude. Climate is also modified by winds which transport heat and moisture from one place to another and by marine currents. Climate determines to a very large extent the character of the animal and vegetable, population of a country or its 'fauna and flora'. In the history, a place is observed with a great many changes of climate, sometimes the era supporting a tropical vegetation and at other times offering a congenial ground for herds of various animals. The alterations in the relative distribution of the masses of land and water account for differences in climate, but often these changes are so extreme that geologists are not able to explain all the phenomena satisfactorily and explanations are to be sought in astronomical causes.

Sun's Distance & Magnitude

During the total eclipses of the Sun around the margin of the disc, are seen various coloured prominences and these hydrogen flames, dart forth in fantastic shapes to the extent of 100 to 150 thousand miles or even to greater distances. Hydrogen gas forms a large portion of the water on the Earth and it is a significant fact that it plays an important part in the constitution of the Sun. The Sun is 92 millions of miles from the Earth and at this inconceivable distance the effects of the solar rays are so powerful that all our phenomena are attributed to their influence. Experiments have shown, the body of the Sun has a large number of metallic and non-metallic elements, and many of them are also found in the composition of the Earth, its minerals, vegetables and animals. The diameter of the Sun is 850,000 miles, its mass is 318,000 times larger than that of the Earth, and the volume is 1,260,000 times more than that of the Earth. From its insignificant size and position the Earth receives less than two thousand millionth part of the total quantity of the Sun's light and heat, and all earthly phenomena must therefore be affected by this extremely minute fraction of solar energy. The mass which makes a man to the mass that forms the globe, so should be the proportion of the Sun's light and heat to call the individual body into a form to the total quantity of his energy, necessary to maintain the globe at the incredible distance of more than 92 millions of miles. If it can be conceived what fraction of the Earth a man is, then that fraction of the less than the two thousandth millionth part of the Sun's energy will be quite enough to bring an individual into existence and destroy him.

Astrology is a Science

Astrology has been very much neglected in recent times and it is regrettable that even the so called educated men judge it, without an effort on their part to know its principles.

Astrology and Medicine are practical sciences and require to be handled as such. The best men studied and believed Astrology would think absurd to bring home charges of ignorance and imposture. No man can pronounce an opinion upon any subject until he has devoted some time for its study and investigation. To laugh at things which men do not take the trouble to know, is the height of folly. Recent scientific researches have shown that many of the Hindu customs were the result of a long and careful study of the sanitary or hygienic principles and not the arbitrary dicta of ignorant and self-designing priests. The meaningless ceremonies and observances were not mere conventionalities which were the result of social or priestly tyranny, but were rules founded on human experience and scientific knowledge. Planets influence all earthly phenomena, but it is difficult to explain or understand the subtleties of those planetary influences without honesty and deep study. I admit it is a very difficult question and no attempt should be made in a primer of this kind to answer it at any considerable length. I shall briefly indicate the direction in which if one takes trouble, one may be able to know more. The question may be considered under three different aspects, (1) Planetary influences on the physical constitution of men, (2) their influence on his intellect, and (3) their influences on him in his life and prospects.

Planets Influences on Human Constitution

I shall consider them in the order I have named. One rotation of the Earth on its own axis constitutes a day and one revolution round the Sun makes a year. The Sun moves on his own axis and is also said to move at a tremendous velocity through space. This double rotation of the Earth and the Sun must account for all the complicated phenomena. There are huge dark spots in the Sun which absorb much of the surrounding light. These are believed to be vast cavities which take away much of the overlying light and heat. These dark spots are common to other planets.

Light and heat comes from the sun and these two physical agents give rise to all phenomena. Cohesion, adhesion, gravitation and chemical attraction are constant and universal forces that control the minutest atom in nature as well as the largest compound brought into existence by their combined or individual action. Evolution theory reveals nothing more than this that all the complex phenomena were called into existence out of the simpler materials and they culminated in the formation of man with his most wonderful intellect. Minerals, Vegetables and Animals have been formed under given physical conditions by the direct influences of the planetary rays. The different eras enunciated by scientists were apparently due to the revolution. In fact, the atmosphere affords one of the most conclusive proofs of the uninterrupted maintenance of existing conditions during enormous periods, but no geologist ventures to extend this doctrine of uniformity beyond the date when fossils appear or to deny that though the laws of Nature are the same, the conditions must have been different directly showing their influences on seasons, waters, altitudes, forests, soils, vegetation and animals and he must be a grand fool who denies these simple and well known facts.

Actions of Sun's Light and Heat

Every object in Nature offers its surface to the action of the Sun's light and heat. The objects are composed of atoms. These atoms enter into an infinite series of combinations, forming parts of organized bodies, vegetable or animal and after discharging their respective functions, they are thrown off again, mixing with the air, the soil, or other organised matter, and again and again running through these rounds of endless physical combinations and dissolutions. When a body is subjected to the action of heat or light, its elements are readily decomposed and its constituent particles are separated, so that many of them combine with other particles and form new substances possessing altogether different properties. Under the Sun's action, atoms are decomposed to their minutest extent possible and every such minute atom feels the force of solar influence. The minuteness of these atoms is a marvel of Nature's work, and passes beyond the conception of man. Take a grain of musk. It will without perceptible diminution, impregnate the atmosphere of a locality for nearly twenty years with its odour; consequently every particle of the atmosphere which produces the sense of odour must contain a certain quantity of the musk. Gold and platinum can be separated into very fine particles, and spun out of incredulous extents. Our skin is tanned by the solar rays. In the same manner, different planetary rays are needed for the development of our different senses, and the minuteness of their work in the scale of creation is simply wonderful.

Planets shine by borrowed light and they are retained in their orbits by gravitation from the Sun. The Sun draws all cosmical materials towards himself; he also imparts to them tremendous velocities. The wonderful energy which matter assumes with the increase of velocity can hardly be believed. Ether which intervenes between the Sun and the Earth has tremendous velocity and all planetary rays which pass through this subtle and mysterious agency, acquire very extraordinary powers. In their onward course, cosmical matters are subjected to the influences of other planets, the patrols of the solar system. In the continual rush of matter, and constant interchange of attendants, we recognize the progress of processes exercising the most potent influence on the welfare of the terrestrial phenomena. Gases are formed by the action of the solar rays and it has been shown by experiment that they are capable of exerting tremendous influences in the formation or destruction of natural objects.

One of the greatest astronomers says "The Sun's rays are the ultimate source of almost every motion which takes place on the surface of the Earth. By its heat are produced all winds, and those disturbances in the electric equilibrium of the atmosphere which give rise to the phenomena of lightning, and probably also to terrestrial action and the aurora. By their vivifying action, vegetables are enabled to draw support from inorganic matter and become in their turn, the supporter of animals and man and the source of those deposits of dynamic efficiency are laid up for human use in our coal strata. By them, waters of the sea are made to circulate in vapour through the air, and irrigate the land producing springs and rivers. By them are produced all disturbances of the chemical equilibrium of the elements of Nature, which by a series of compositions and decompositions, give rise to new products and originate a transfer of materials. Even though they show degradation of the solid constituents on the surface in which its chief geological change consists of, it is almost entirely due on one hand to the abrasion of wind or rain and the alteration of heat and frost and on the other, to the continual heating of sea waves agitated by winds, the results of solar radiation. The effect of oceanic currents (mainly originating in that influence) though slight in abrasion is powerful in diffusing and transporting the matter abraded and when we consider the immense transfer of matter so produced, the increase of pressure over large spaces in the bed of the ocean and the diminution over corresponding portions of the land, we are not at a loss to perceive, how the elastic force of subterranean fires, thus repressed on the one hand and released on the other, may break forth in points where the resistance is barely adequate to their retention and thus bring the phenomena of even volcanic activity under the general law of solar influence. I have said enough to a thinking mind to show that we are directly under the influence of the planetary rays and that every phenomenon we witness around us, is the direct result of such influences. Men are incessantly acted upon by invisible and inconceivable forces and their influences are perceptible to even the most ignorant. It is surely no sin to believe what one feels. Physically therefore, it is plain that man is under the direct influence of planetary rays as all terrestrial forces are controlled by the solar energy.

Coming to the second division, I shall say a few words. Psychological niceties distinguish between mind and body. It is broad enough to the ordinary mind.

If "mind" is something not the result of birth, breeding, education and surroundings, then its presence in the human body must be credited to the unknown hand, to which any name may be applied. But if we have to consider our "will" as the result of birth, breeding, education and surroundings, we can easily trade its work in the conditions under which it is called into existence. Sensation and feelings are located in the brain and these are centered there by means of external impressions carried through the nervous system springing from the head and branching through the spinal column. Sexual union is necessary for propagation and the vital essence is formed out of the food we take. This active principle of reproduction cannot be had without the ordinary conditions of life. After sexual union with man and conception, the woman requires greater nourishment and care than before. It is clear that food, climate and other physical conditions become indispensable for the development of the foetus. After certain stages by the influence of planetary rays, the babe is thrown out and takes a separate and individual existence. It is material, therefore, to see where the child is born, for much of its future success depends upon its surroundings in the commencement. Both before and after its birth the child as well as its parents are under the direct influence of the Sun and his attendant planets. There is the brain undeveloped and ready to receive impressions to be stored up for future purposes of reference. Astrologers place the Soul under the direct influence of the Sun while the mind is credited to the lunar effects. Planets in their reflections of the solar rays show a marked difference. The air is the same all over the world, but as it is considerably affected by the contact of local objects, so also do the rays of the Sun, undergo a change with their contact with other planets. They give something of their own and take something from the objects with which they come in contact.

When the solar light is refracted, the spectra contain seven different colours, and their heating powers are different, diminishing towards the violet and increasing towards the red. At the green part of the band, the effects of the two extremes seems to be perfectly neutralised. Solar rays produce considerable changes in the appearance and constitution of many substances. Idiots and lunatics are considerably affected on new moon and full moon days. A needle before a magnet shows an invisible cause of motion. We know it as magnetism, but we do not know why that phenomenon is produced. In a similar way, electricity is generated by contact of certain substances. The greater the nervous energy of a man, the greater is the will force in him. It is not the quantity of flesh and blood that make a great man a but the quantity and quality of the brain stuff that make him, great man. Mind is affected by the surrounding phenomena. Sunstrokes, mirages, heated atmospheres, poisonous gases, the luxuriant growth of the tropics, the stunted shrubberies of the frigids, the exhibition of vitality among the lowest forms of insects, the storing in of electrical currents among the marine animals, the great virtues of the medicinal herbs, the powers of the plants and the animals in the selection and assimilation of their food, the convulsion of the Earth and celestial phenomena; all these directly affect the human mind. It is stupidity to deny their influences.

The different types of mankind are the striking illustrations of their influences. When the Earth is called into its present shape by their solar influences, where is the logic of showing that bodies on its surface are not affected by them. Changes in the thermometer record changes in human mind. A trifling change in weather through solar causes brings on neuralgia, headache, bronchitis, sore eyes, fever, smallpox, cholera, dysentery, plague and a host of other diseases, too numerous to detail. Could there be mind unaffected by climatic changes? Changes in the compositions of the solar rays considerably affect the flora and the fauna of a country. War mania is a striking illustration of the planetary influences.

Ever calculating and selfish to a degree, the poor mortal, rushes on to a work of destruction, which very often ends in the annihilation of families, nay villages, towns and even nations.

When evil planets aspect each other and are devoid of beneficial aspects or conjunctions, nations plunge into war most headlong and perish by thousands and hundreds of thousands. The mental calibre of each individual is determined by the quality and quantity of his brain which affect his prospects in life and which is directly under the influence of planets. Whether the mind is placed in man by God or is the result of birth and surroundings, in either case, it must be granted that it is directly affected by the natural phenomena which surrounds it. A reference to the world's history will show that the greatest men died generally on or before new moon days. If a person has strong will power, he is sure to rise far above his surroundings, however humble they may be. Biographies of eminent men amply confirm the statement. A favourable conjunction of the planets rises a man far above his birth and condition, while an unfavourable combination brings him down to the lowest grade even if he chances to be the son of a mighty monarch. Forces minute to a degree, produce wonderful changes in Nature and they emanate from the Sun and his attendant planets. Moon represents mind and the slightest obliquity in her rays produces marked differences in his mental calibre. The art by which we calculate these forces constitutes the subject power of Astrology and the symbols are used with a view to show their results. The time of birth and the position of the planets then, as well as their revolutions from day to day, from month to month and from year to year, must be taken into consideration in determining the results of their influences, combinations and permutations of these planets, zodiacal signs, constellation and their divisions which produces an endless variety in the life of man and if properly worked out, can account for all the terrestrial and celestial phenomena by which men are surrounded. It is clear therefore, that mind is strengthened or weakened by man's surroundings and the climatic changes which he is subjected to.

The different temperaments of the various nations, positively prove that, whatever may be the final source of the human 'mind', it can never be averred that it is not influenced by food, climate, heredity, occupation and the society in which it finds itself. If the sun is the final source for all electrical currents and they represent all nervous energy in man, then the influence of the Sun on man and his mind is thoroughly demonstrated.

I now come to the 3rd division and conclude this Introduction with a few observations on that point. The Sun sends all natural forces. Electricity and magnetism comes from him. Electricity is of two kinds, positive and negative. Nature is pervaded by this great physical agent. Contact of silver and sulphuric acid gives us positive while zinc and sulphuric acid produces negative electricity. Electricities of the same nature repel each other, while those of the opposite kind attract each other. Herein lies the secret of man's success and failure. In some objects positive preponderates while in others negative takes the ascendancy. Sometimes, under certain given physical conditions these change their sides suddenly; positive becoming negative and *vice versa*. Nervous currents become the most important factors in man. He could do nothing without them. Physical and mental causes determine the preponderance of the electrical currents in the parents, hence also in the child. In some places, plants and animals have peculiar tendencies to store in large quantities positive or negative electricities and this will be marked in particular seasons or on particular occasions of days. Hindus pick up medicinal herbs on new moon days falling on Sundays and under certain constellations, certain plants are also said to possess the virtues of subjugating the wills of other persons or *Rajavasyam or Tanavasyam.* Success means influence with men of business and bringing them to our ways of thinking and doing. The phenomena is thus explained scientifically. A man has 'x' will power and goes to a man with '2x' will power. The law of nature is that the stronger shall conquer the weaker. Matter attracts in proportion to its mass. The '2x' man will have to be subjugated by a superior mental force. The greater the magnetic power, the greater the attraction. By keeping herbs of great virtue with him a person gains more than '2x' power and thus subjugates him who now appears the weaker party. Mesmerism is based upon this principle of subduing weak wills by stronger mental concentration. The contact of people of higher will force with other, of an inferior type is always injurious to the former as by the nature of electrical currents, they are always induced from the great body to the smaller, something like water flowing from a higher level to a lower. The greater the possession of electricity, the greater the success and personal influence of the man. The less the possession of will power, the less are the chances of success to the person.

Men with superior merits are not honoured in some places where fools are honoured. The astrologer tells the places which are good for their business, where they will meet with ready success and also with what kind of people. This is nothing, but a determination of the different forces working within and without human bodies and these are expressed as so many symbols in Astrology. Officers, kings, professors, ladies, gentlemen, animals, and in fact every kind of object has its own favourite or favourites and such favouritism is the result of electrical or magnetic currents. When two positively electrified persons meet, they hate each other and this means failure and loss. When oppositely electrified persons meet, there is friendship and this means success and gain. The directions, times and classes of persons and individuals must be known, as they can be, by Astrology and then men can have success.

There is an irresistible temptation to love or hate a person when he is positively or negatively electrified. Human tastes, on which depends their success in life, are examples of the same unaccountable influences. Sometimes they loose and sometimes they gain by them. When there are so many forces at work, sometimes in union, and sometimes against each other, the results from such working will also be favourable or otherwise, according to the nature of the powers which produce them. Friends quarrel with each other when their electrical currents change and enemies become friends again when there are similar changes in their influences. The successes and failure of men were keenly watched by the intelligent classes of all times and were associated with the appearances of certain stars, combinations of planets, and their revolution round the Sun. The Sun shining through his millions and billions of rays, affects all bodies, all minds and all prospects in life. He makes a man courageous or timid as he sheds a greater or less influence on the person in question. Solar rays enter the human body and produce health in some, disease in others. Changes in the weather produce changes in the creation and destruction of minerals, vegetables and animals. All these are controlled by the solar rays.

Disturbances in the jovian globe have a direct effect upon the magnetic currents in the solar disc, and these again are directly connected with terrestrial magnetism. It is well established by careful observations, that the flora and the fauna are vegetation and animals in any locality are directly affected by the magnetic currents there and thus it is clearly seen that the planetary influences are exercising their powers on everything which we find on the earth. The ancient Scholars had a thorough knowledge of the effects of magnetic currents, and even their precepts in religious matters, show their unmistakable desire to improve physical health and mental vigour. In the change of opinions, dress, manners, customs, countries, wives, religion, modes of life, tastes and education, the electrical currents are seen playing the most important part. Certain nerves in the brain are identified, with certain tastes, their undue development at the cost of other nerves, makes men pursue a particular line of conduct. Nervous currents are identified with electrical currents. Electrical currents are under the direct influence of the planetary rays and these produce development or depression according to certain given physical conditions. Whether the ancients had such deep knowledge in the physical sciences, is doubted by some one-sided writers who at best get a second hand information and fill up the gaps with their own unjustifiable fancies. The knowledge of the ancient Hindus in mathematics, astronomy, logic, grammar, medicine, psychology, philosophy, mechanics and religion has never been surpassed by the ancient or modern nations. The fabulous cycles of years given by the Hindu astronomers of late have been receiving greater and greater confirmation at the hands of the astronomer, chemist, physicist, geologist and psychologist, while the eras named by the half named, by the half informed and Biblical writers have been held to be utterly worthless for scientific references. They were highly intelligent and practical. They never said or did anything without purpose. The *sutras* are most suggestive and useful.

The hair splitting speculative philosophers of the East had a very good knowledge of the natural laws which controlled them, and were certainly superior to the self-conceited, and ill-informed philosophers of the West. Foreign conquest did a good deal of mischief to our ancient arts and sciences and this was specially the case during the time of the Mohammed ascendancy. In judging of past civilisation we have to make very large allowances for the destroying hand of time and the incessant changes which are taking place from various causes. If there is anything sublime in this world, it is Astrology and the following qualifications have`been laid down as indispensable for successful prediction: -

1. No mean motives
2. Contentment
3. High proficiency in mathematics
4. Linguistic command
5. Great intelligence
6. A knowledge of the times and circumstances
7. A thorough knowledge of the astrological technicalities
8. Honesty and sincerity
9. Truthfulness
10. Proper initiation

I can say that these qualifications are not commonly met with and those who profess to know Astrology know very little of it. This is as it ought not to be. Much uncertainty and failure result from a want of these qualifications, and want of state support and sympathy keeps away the best men in the field from taking up the study of Astrology as a paying or honourable profession.

There are some cheats who predict most faithfully the past, but fail most miserably in their future predictions. Such men are generally successful and carry away large sums of money. This must be put an end to. To know the feature has ever been the greatest ambition of man, and this knowledge can be safely acquired by studying Astrology. It is easy to ask a lot of questions, but not so easy to answer them by the light of known scientific principles, which from their imperfections are not able to explain many facts known and recorded as true by the most learned of the ancients.

Many who consult their horoscopes forget that they have to pay for the work they expect the astrologer to do. This conduct on the part of educated and intelligent men is highly reprehensible, and must be condemned for two reasons, (1) because it considerably lowers the efficiency of astrology as a paying profession, and (2) because it makes the astrologers careless and indifferent in their calculations and predictions, since they see no sufficient remuneration for very serious mental work.

Astrology like Medicine is a practicable science and must be useful all along. Astrology will be perfectly useless when the predictions are not fulfilled. It is useless to get good written prescription when the medicine gives men no relief. The results in medical science are far from being satisfactory. It has been encouraged by State authority and has been therefore called a science although there are greater failures than in Medicines in Astrology in spite of all neglect. For enormous sums spent on medical establishment, the percentage of cures is positively discouraging. Fever, leprosy, smallpox, cholera, dysentery, and consumption are not properly explained and successfully treated. Every medical man, whether he cures or kills, will have his bills paid in preference to others. In my humble experience and observance, nearly half the numbers that present themselves in the hospitals go back without relief, and if more cures are effected than the low percentage, it is by the general prescription of *aqua pura* and by the help of mother Nature and not by the skill of the medical profession. Medicine is praised beyond its desert. If there is more sickness than ought to be, it is because medical men publish such books and by reading them make men sick while they really are not so, by working on their fancy or imagination. While every noble attempt has been made to raise medicine to the level of a science, nothing worthy of record has been done to test Astrology. The ancients studied and has tested Astrology. The ancients studied the two together and found out that one could not be satisfactorily understood without the aid of the other. Astrology has stood its ground in spite of the hostile attacks to root it out altogether and its predictions are not such as to create genuine dislike in the minds of those who have really taken pains to master its details. Some say that a knowledge of the future is bad as it damps their spirits and unnerves one from further exertions. This is not a closed question. In cases of incurable diseases, patients know that they are subjected to forms of diseases before which the medical men simply blink, but they do not die because they are not subjected to them or because medical science has declared them to be beyond its sphere of cure.

When such incurable diseases set in, the doctor cannot pollute his life by making false statements, that the patient is not suffering from them, and that the patient will live for a long time. What difference then does it make between the statement of an astrologer who says that the planetary period is bad and therefore he must suffer from it unless he takes proper remedial measures for averting those evil influences and that of the doctor who says that the patient must shift for himself as best as he could, since medical science has not explained even the nature of such a disease. Sudden dangers, it is true kill some, but let them only be smoothly informed of it beforehand; the sorrow distributes itself and makes its keenness as little felt as possible. Necessity is the mother of invention. Human genius is stimulated under great adversities, and when persons know that there is evil before them, they will do their best to find means to over come it. Human nature is very plausible and accommodates itself to the exigencies of every case. 'South Sea Bubbles' often burst, but men concerned in such affairs are not drowned at once in sorrow and die.

An astrologer interprets the language of the planets by the symbols used and predicts the future events by their light. Insurance Companies warn men of their uncertain deaths. Every man of sense must be prepared to meet death, misery or the loss of those who are dear and near to him. It is a good saying. 'Hope for the best, but be prepared for the worst'.

If a person is not prepared to meet the stern realities of his life, but fancies that death and misery dare not invade his homestead, let no such coward ever consult his horoscope. Men with halters round their necks and death floating before their lusterless eyes, have been known to show utter disregard for life and if the predictions of an astrologer are more horrible than the death sentences of the life-taking judges, let such timid men never consult their fate. Where ignorance is bliss, it is folly to be wise. Knowledge of every kind always destroys our peace of mind by creating one thousand and one doubts and if it is not desirable to cultivate it for this, then it might be conveniently sacrificed for the so called peace of mind which is nothing, but ignorance and guilt rolled together and which is not prepared to see the light of knowledge and wisdom.

If there are people who get dispirited by such predictions, who being by their very nature weak and useless, could do nothing that is noble or useful, there are many who, emboldened by hopeful or adverse prediction, exert themselves tenfold and do more good work than they could have done without them. There could possibly be no loss by knowing our future by making or attempting to make suitable arrangements to meet it and to cultivate our *"will force"* to a greater extent so that if it is possible, as it is always possible to overcome all evil influences by strong will force and other remedies prescribed in the Hindu Shastras. We may try to counteract or control the natural forces which guide our future and under whose influence we have been called into existence. Would it not prove a grand acquisition to our store of knowledge to know whence we have come, what we will be and where we will go? Can such a grand science be called stupid or absurd? From the idle experiments and investigations of alchemists in the middle ages, arose the beautiful science of Chemistry, Physics and Medicine. Metaphysics, Philosophy and many other subjects give men no practicable help and their study adds no comfort to their material enjoyment. But the intellectual treat they afford them, compensates for all the labour a person bestows upon them. The intellectual treat in Astrology is the greatest and richest one can imagine and as it affects human interests working in a million different ways for their accomplishment, it is worthy of pursuit by the greatest as well as the meanest of mankind.

I shall close my Introduction by quoting a few marks made by an eminent writer on the intellectual greatness of our ancient writers, who, gigantic as they were in other branches of learning, did not consider the study of Astrology detrimental to the progress of their nation or inconsistent with their avowed principles of utility. Astrological predictions did not damp their spirits and the few monuments of their greatness and splendour spared to posterity by the destructive hand of time, show unmistakably that they were not only the greatest thinkers, but also were the greatest actors the world had ever seen. The writer says "I have called the mind of this (Hindu) race... the Brain of the East." The latest philosophical and religious system lay prefigured in the depths of this Hindu brain. It created one of the most artistic languages and one of the richest literatures in the world. It complied elaborate Law codes in large numbers and besides its voluminous Bibles gathered immense treasures of sacred lore, ritual, philosophical and devotional. Its poetic productivity was prodigious. Its great epics Ramayana and Mahabaratha glow with luxuriance of imagery which contrasts with the Illiad or Aenied, as the stupendous vegetation of India differs from that of Italy or Greece. All that this colossal people have dreamed or done in philosophy, mythology, ethics, imagination or didactic thought, is here transmuted into song.

The earlier Hindus had well organised Governments, much lauded by the Greek writers for the wise and thoughtful manner in which the interests of trade and agriculture were protected, the wants of strangers, as of the sick and needy supplied, and the defence of the state secured. India has at all times been famous for its domestic and foreign trade. In more than one epoch, the resources of India, natural and industrial as well as intellectual, have made the wealth of great Empires. Its delicate tissues, its marvellous colours and dyes, its porcelains, its work in metals and stones, its dainty essences and perfumes, have not only been the wonder and delight of Europe, but in no sight degree helped in the revival of art. The intellectual life of India was profoundly felt throughout the ancient world. They have only applied Algebra to Astronomy and Geometry, but geometry to the demarcation of algebraic rules. The decimal system was developed in India as a speculative calculus so earnestly that special names were given to every power in an ascending scale of enormous reach. The fifty third power of ten was taken as a unit and on this new base another scale of numbers rose till a figure was reached consisting of this unity followed by four hundred and twenty one zeroes.

Aryabhatta, the greatest astronomer and mathematician in the fourth century B.C. determined very closely the relation of the diameter of a circle to the circumstance and applied it to the measurement of the Earth. The physicians were skilful enough to win the admiration of the Greeks. Aryabhatta appears to have reached by independent observations about the knowledge of the Earth's movement on its axis, and to have availed himself of the science of his time, in calculating the procession of the equinoxes and the length of the orbital times of planets. In whatsoever, concerning the study of words or forms the Hindus have always been at home anticipating the Greeks and accomplishing more at the outset of their career than the Semitic races did in two thousand years. We have to remember that this praise of the Hindus comes from a foreigner, who at best has only a very superficial view of the whole range of Hindu Knowledge, transmitted to him through many perverted channels. Our social tall-talk reformers should remember that before they open their mouths to censure Hindu sciences, they have to show to the world that they possess enough capacity to understand what is contained in the sacred books of the East if they mean to command any public attention at all. In its absence we must only pity the simple fools who talk because they think they know how to talk, and who unfortunately have no judgement to call their own.

I shall here say something about the remedial measures and close my introduction. Man is the crowning glory of terrestrial creation. In his body and head are found machinery and construction, the finest ever invented. In fact the wonders of genius are still a great wonder to itself. Psychology puzzles man more than anything else. Yoga and Gnana are two departments wherein are laid the precepts for the evolution of a power before which the greatest natural forces, discovered by man sink to insignificance. Mental power is the greatest because nothing equal to it has ever been discovered. The power of holding breath, the process of introspection and the practices of yoga are mysteries which are utterly unknown to the Western sciences. It is not speculation that plays any part here, but real self-denial and determined practice. These are unknown to orientalists who make much of their superficial knowledge of Hindu Sciences and Literature.

There are two powers in man, the human or physical and the spiritual or Brahmashakti. Lifting of the veils of ignorance, will take inner man to a higher spiritual elevation where he sees things altogether in a different light. The physical composition is affected by the *Pancha Mahabootas* not elements as misrepresented by Sanscrities, but the mental or divine which is above their jurisdiction. Electricity combines the grosser and the finer natures in mysterious bond. The finer is the essence of the grosser. Therefore, a smaller quantity of the finer will be able to put down or cancel a larger quantity of the grosser. By our mental determination and strength, we mostly overcome the extensive physical temptation to which we are subjected. A man sees a splendid woman. The whole body of the woman offers his whole body a tremendous temptation. He does not know the extent of his mind, but minute as it may be, if it is only divine or moral, he at once rejects the woman and even will get the strength of mind and loathe her presence. A divine man is persecuted and consigned to flames. The physical plains are excruciating, but his powerful mind rejects to beg any help or change its conviction.

The sense for duty urges many to lay down their lives under the most distressing circumstances. All these show that the finer is always more valuable than the grosser. With such a mind in man, he can do wonders as he has done. The abnegations which the greatest Hindus have subjected themselves to, could never be practiced by the materialistic West which is more after the flesh than after the mind. The planets are indicators of previous Karma. It is absurd to think that men suddenly jump over the world in their present shape at one make. There must have been various stages of developments. In equalities, in physique, in mind, and in prospects, often for no fault of ours, results prove the *Karma theory.* When previous Karmic results are indicated by planets, they blind the *Sthula sharira,* physical body and not the *jeeva* or soul, although the latter is found in and attached to the body. There is no fatalism that man must suffer for what he has done. He has some independence, as every grade of government service has some discretion given to it. A karmic result is shown by the planetary combinations, Dashas and

Bhukties. Here they do not prevent exertion on the part of the soul or jeeva.

The sun shines and heats a surface. He does not invite or prohibit persons or animals to come or go from that place, it is something like this. Men may reap the fruits of their past karma or overcome them by their self-exertions. The Karma is binding only to a reasonable extent. Where Brahmashakti develops, Karmashakti recedes and may be finally overcome. If this were not so, the whole world would be a void and man a purposeless being. Vedantha, Yoga, Mantra and Vaidya Sastras have been framed by Maharishis to enable man to grapple with his terrestrial and Karmic difficulties and overcome them by developing Brahmashakti. Processes are laid down based upon heat, sound, light and electrical vibrations to avert the evil influences of planets on the grosser natures of mankind. It is therefore, absolutely necessary for every man to know that he is his own *cut-throat* when he neglects to be profited by opportunities. The above named sciences enable one to ward off the evil and court the good. The skill of the astrologer consists in exactly knowing the intensity of danger and prescribing remedies to meet it. Sound causes us pain and pleasure. The vedic swara is based upon a minute knowledge of this important principle. Heart increases or decreases sound and as all rays indicate certain degrees of heart, hence vibration of sound it is necessary to find out whence pain comes and what remedies counter would remove painful sensations. This is a difficult problem and cannot be satisfactorily discussed in an elementary book like the one under preparation.

The subject is a vast one and requires volumes to be written on it. I shall here recapitulate the principal points once more so that the attentive reader might see, what scientific grounds he has, for holding astrology as true and how he could meet the silly objection of those, who out of ignorance put any question they have in their heads. All the planets including the Earth revolve round the Sun. The Earth gets infinitesimally small quantity of the Solar energy and this has been shown to be sufficient to account for all the terrestrial phenomena. Light brings heat, magnetism and electricity Gravitation is universal as also the forces of cohesion, adhesion and chemical attraction. Solar energy influences everything on the surface of the Earth. Oceans, atmosphere and marine currents are under the influence of the solar rays. Man is the result of previous forces working under definite laws with such local modifications as are found to be necessary in each individual case. His physical constitution is under their direct influence, because the seed that produced him, the bed in which he was nourished, the food he takes, the clothing he wears, the water he drinks and the air he breathes are entirely the results of the Sun's rays working in Nature in their own inscrutable ways.

The nervous system is greatly affected by the time, place, seed, food, climate and other conditions of life and intellect is solely dependent upon the quantity and quality of the brain cells derived from those sources. Our vision would be worse than useless, had there been no solar light and similarly our other senses, each of which has been made to work under the direct influence of a particular planet. Planets shine by borrowed light from the solar rays and add something of their own and thus influence mankind in various ways. The Moon exerts great influences on our minds. Lunatics, idiots and mad men exhibit marked changes on full moon and new moon days and sick people pass restless nights. The greatest men of the world believed in astrology and would not have done so, had it not been practically demonstrated. Electricity is the great physical agent which pervades through the Universe and has been known to produce the strongest phenomena. The intellect of man is the result of the nervous currents passing through the human frame and forming what is familiarly called mind or will. Whatever *"mind"* may be, it cannot remain for any length of time unaffected by its surroundings and the food and climate are important factors in the determination of our mind. It is therefore, under the direct influence of the Sun's light and heat and might have been called into existence by their combined chemical action.

The greater the solar influence, the greater the nervous energy in man.

There are two kinds of electricities – positive and negative, both directly taking their source in the solar energy. Similar electricities repel other while opposite kinds attract one another. The preponderance in Natural or electrical currents of the positive or negative kind, depend upon thousand circumstances which cannot be detailed here. Rivers, mountains, lakes, elevated grounds, rocks, forests, hamlets, village, towns, cities, and even individual houses possess sometimes, of storing in large quantities of positive or negative electricities, due to causes working previously there under certain given physical conditions. They suddenly change their sides, positive becoming negative and vice versa. Our tastes, our success, our failure and our energy depend on the electrical currents.

Inconceivable fractions of the Sun's light and heat are sufficient to produce the greatest perceptible changes in Nature. It is seen what minute fraction of the solar force is enough to keep the Earth as it is, with all its flora and its fauna, and how we have to conceive, an inconceivable fraction of this infinitesimally small fraction of the solar power that is needed to bring an individual into existence and destroy him again for redistribution in nature. The revolutions of the planets round the Sun; their absorbing and reflecting powers of light and heat, the rotation of the Sun on his own axis, the presence or absence of huge dark spots darting forth vast flames of hydrogen gas from the body of the sun for thousands of miles, and their fall again upon his disc, the passage through space of the Sun with all his attendant planets at a tremendous velocity, the nearness or distance of the Earth from the Sun in her revolutions round him, these and many other causes most of which are not known to us, must account satisfactorily for the different historical periods, changes in social life, political convulsions, difference in morality, alterations in taste, intellectual developments, creation of new species, extinction of old animals, distribution of the masses of land and water, and in fact for every other things for which we find no records in the past or no parallel in the future. The gigantic minds of the ancients were sufficiently large enough to store in vast quantities of knowledge of all kinds and possessing, as they did an acutely critical turn of mind, they could not have been deceived by the tissue of an elaborate system of falsehood invented by the self interested priests and pandits. The degradation of the science of astrology has been chiefly due to the political convulsions, the ignorance and greed of astrologers, the anxiety of person who recklessly consult them, and the difficult nature of the science which requires for its success, profound knowledge and patient research. Truth was held in the highest veneration by our ancestors and the sin of desertion from its sacred shrine by the modern astrologers has been visited upon them. The mean jealously which characterises the modern Hindu and his unwillingness to see others making rapid intellectual advance, have not been without their poisonous fruit and if astrology has not been as successful in its predictions as it ought to have been, the fault lies more with the professors into whose hands it has fallen than to any radical inaccuracies found in its countless pages. Experience must be the backbone of every science and handful of such is worth more than cartloads of theoretical knowledge. My works have always been received with very great favour by the educated public and this fact encourages me to labour more in the same field and make the subject as simple as it is possible for me to do. I am a self-taught man and had no difficulty to master its technicalities. I hope this primer will pave the way for readers, who take the interest in this subject and who are anxious to know more of astrological science. If the readers find it interesting and instructive, I consider myself well rewarded for the trouble I have taken in completing this small work.

B. SURYANARAIN RAO

❖❖❖

Learn Yourself VEDIC ASTROLOGY *IN 15 DAYS*

CHAPTER - 1

YEARS, AYANAS, RUTHUS AND MONTHS

The Hindu cycle contains 60 lunar years. They are:

1.	Prabhava	1987 -	88	**22.**	Sarwadhari	2008 -	09
2.	Vibhava	1988 -	89	**23.**	Virodhi	2009 -	10
3.	Shukla	1989 -	90	**24.**	Vikruti	2010 -	11
4.	Pramoduta	1990 -	91	**25.**	Khara	2011 -	12
5.	Prajotpatti	1991 -	92	**26.**	Nandana	2012 -	13
6.	Angirasa	1992 -	93	**27.**	Vijaya	2013 -	14
7.	Srimukha	1993 -	94	**28.**	Jaya	2014 -	15
8.	Bhava	1994 -	95	**29.**	Manmatha	2015 -	16
9.	Yuva	1995 -	96	**30.**	Durmukhi	2016 -	17
10.	Dhatu	1996 -	97	**31.**	Hevilambi	2017 -	18
11.	Ishwara	1997 -	98	**32.**	Vilambi	2018 -	19
12.	Bahudanya	1998 -	99	**33.**	Vikari	2019 -	20
13.	Pramadhi	1999 -	2000	**34.**	Sharwari	2020 -	21
14.	Vikrama	2000 -	2001	**35.**	Plava	2021 -	22
15.	Vishu	2001 -	02	**36.**	Shubhakrutu	2022 -	23
16.	Chitrabhanu	2002 -	03	**37.**	Shobhakrutu	2023 -	24
17.	Swabhanu	2003 -	04	**38.**	Krodhi	2024 -	25
18.	Tharana	2004 -	05	**39.**	Vishwavasu	2025 -	26
19.	Parthiva	2005 -	06	**40.**	Parabhava	2026 -	27
20.	Vyaya	2006 -	07	**41.**	Plavanga	2027 -	28
21.	Sarwajitu	2007 -	08	**42.**	Kilaka	2028 -	29

43.	Soumya	2029 -	30	53.	Siddaharti	2039 -	40
44.	Sadharana	2030 -	31	54.	Roudri	2040 -	41
45.	Virodhikrutu	2031 -	32	55.	Durmathi	2041 -	42
46.	Paridhavi	2032 -	33	56.	Dundubhi	2042 -	43
47.	Pramadicha	2033 -	34	57.	Rudhirodgari	2043 -	44
48.	Ananda	2034 -	35	58.	Rakthakshi	2044 -	45
49.	Rakshasa	2035 -	36	59.	Krodhana	2045 -	46
50.	Nala	2036 -	37	60.	Akshaya	1986 -	87
51.	Pingala	2037 -	38	61.	Prabhava	2046 -	47
52.	Kalayukti	2038 -	39				

Note: Subtract 60 from the current year to get previous set of sixty years cycle.

Ayanas (Solstices)

The Hindu year is divided into two equal parts, each of which is called an Ayana. They are **1.** Uttarayana (Winter Solstice) when the Sun moves in a north direction and **2.** Dakshinayana (Summer Solstice) when the Sun moves in a south direction.

Uttaryana has six solar months, viz.

1. Capricorn—Makara **2.** Aquarius—Kumbha **3.** Pisces—Meena **4.** Aries—Mesha **5.** Taurus—Vrishabha **6.** Gemini—Mithuna.

Dakshinayana has six solar months, viz.

1. Cancer—Kataka **2.** Leo—Simha **3.** Virgo—Kanya **4.** Libra—Tula **5.** Scorpio—Vrischika **6.** Sagittarius—Dhanus.

Months

The twelve lunar months are named as follows:—

1. Chaitra **2.** Vyshakha **3.** Jyeshta **4.** Ashadha **5.** Sravana **6.** Bhadrapada **7.** Ashwija **8.** Karttika **9.** Mrigasira **10.** Pushya **11.** Makha **12.** Phalguna.

Seasons

There are six Ruthus (or seasons, as different from four seasons, amongst the Westerners) each containing two lunar months and they are:

1. Vasantha—Chaitra and Vyshaka, when the trees and plants blossom.
2. Greeshma—Jyeshta and Ashadha, when there is a good deal of wind.
3. Varsha—Sravana and Bhadrapada, when it is a rainy season.
4. Sharat—Ashwija and Karttika, when there will be fruits.
5. Himantha—Mrigasira and Pushya, when there will be cold.
6. Shishira—Makha and Phalguna, when trees and plants put forth leaves.

Reasons for Names of Months

The star on the full moon day of the lunar month gives the name to that month. Thus in Chaitra, the star Chaitra falls on the full moon day. In Vyshaka, the constellation Vishaka rules on the full moon day. In Jyeshta, the star Jyeshta comes on Pournima (full moon) and so on for other months.

Zodiacal Signs, Planets and Constellations

There are nine Planets:

1. Sun, **2.** Moon, **3.** Mars, **4.** Mercury, **5.** Jupiter, **6.** Venus, **7.** Saturn, **8.** Dragon's Head, **9.** Dragon's Tail.

Their Sanskrit equivalents and Western symbols are:

Planet	Symbol	Sanskrit names			
Sun	☉	Ravi	Aaditya	Surya	Bhanu
Moon	☽	Chandra	Soma	Indu	Sitarasmi
Mars	♂	Mangala	Kuja	Bhouma	Vakra
Mercury	☿	Budha	Induputra	Somaja	Vit
Jupiter	♃	Guru	Brihaspathi	Jeeva	Suri

Planet	Symbol	Sanskrit names			
Venus	♀	Shukra	Bhargava	Jeeva	Suri
Saturn	♄	Shani	Manda	Pangu	Ravija
Dragon's Head	☊	Rahu	Thama	Abi	Agu
Dragon's Tail	☋	Ketu	Dhwaja	Sikhi	

The planets move along the celestial path (ecliptic) which is marked by 27 constellations or clusters of stars. The planets move from west to east, while the Bhuchakra or the Zodiac of Light marked by the twenty-seven constellations, moves from east to west. In astronomy, we have to unlearn many of our infantile ideas, and learn truths which appear radically different from our popular conceptions.

Names of Constellations or nakshatras

1. Ashwini — 3 stars resembling a horse's face
2. Bharani — 3 stars resembling a female sexual organ
3. Krittika — 6 stars like a razor
4. Rohini — 5 stars resembling a car
5. Mrigasira — 3 stars like a human head
6. Arudra — 1 star like a coral head
7. Punarvasu — 5 stars like a potter's wheel
8. Pushya — 3 stars resembling a blood-sucker
9. Aslesha — 6 stars like a serpent
10. Makha — 5 stars like a palanquin
11. Poorvaphalguni — 2 stars resembling human eyes
12. Uttaraphalguni — 2 stars like eyes
13. Hasta — 5 stars like human fingers
14. Chitra — 1 star like a pearl
15. Swathi — 1 star like a sapphire
16. Visakha — 5 stars like a potter's wheel

17. Anuradha — 3 stars resembling an umbrella
18. Jyeshta — 3 stars resembling an umbrella
19. Moola — 5 stars like a crouching lion
20. Poorvashada — 2 stars each, forming a square
21. Uttarashada — 2 stars each, forming a square
22. Sravana — 3 stars like an arrow
23. Dhanishta — 3 stars like a man's head
24. Satabisha — 100 stars resembling a flower
25. Poorvabhadra — 2 stars each forming the legs of a cot
26. Uttarabhadra — 2 stars each forming the legs of a cot
27. Revati — 3 stars like a fish

Each of these constellations is divided into four quarters or padas and we have 27 × 4 = 108 padas comprising the whole of the Zodiac. Each pada gets 3½ degrees.

The Zodiac

The Zodiac is a celestial circle divided into 360 equal parts called Bhagas or degrees. It is divided into twelve equal divisions called Rashis or signs. The first point of Mesha, which is the beginning of the Zodiac, is also the first point of Ashwini. The twelve signs, their Symbols and Sanskrit equivalents are:

1.	Aries	♈	Ram	Mesha	Aja
2.	Taurus	♉	Bull	Vrishabha	Vrisha
3.	Gemini	♊	Twins	Mithuna	Nriyuk
4.	Cancer	♋	Crab	Kataka	Kulira
5.	Leo	♌	Lion	Simha	Hari
6.	Virgo	♍	Virgin	Kanya	Angana
7.	Libra	♎	Balance	Tula	Vanik
8.	Scorpio	♏	Scorpion	Vrischika	Kita
9.	Sagittarius	♐	Centaur	Dhanus	Chapa
10.	Capricorn	♑	Crocodile	Makara	Mriga
11.	Aquarius	♒	Water-bearer	Kumbha	Hridroga
12.	Pisces	♓	Fish	Meena	Antya

Each of these signs is composed of nine quarters or padas of stars and we have

$\frac{27\times 4}{12}$ = 9 padas. A study of the map attached at the end of the work is strongly recommended. It will help the reader understand the following pages.

Each of the signs therefore gets 30 degrees and as a sign is composed of 9 quarters, each pada gets 30/9 or 3 1/3 degrees. Fractions of these must be found out by elaborate calculations. A good knowledge in Mathematics is indispensable for proficiency in Astrology and those who are not familiar with figures, will never be able to make much progress for all calculations. The Zodiac must be commenced from Aries or Mesha, and it is called the Adi sign unless the contrary appears from the context. This must be specially remembered as otherwise the reader will fall into great confusion in the study of the astrological principles. In horoscopes planets are usually placed from the Lagna or birth sign, when referring to Bhavas or significations (Houses).

❖❖❖

CHAPTER - 2

PLANETARY NATURES, STRENGTHS, ETC.

Good and Evil Planets

Planets are good or evil as their influences are favourable or unfavourable to mankind. Good planets are Jupiter, Venus, well associated Mercury and Full Moon.

Evil planets are Sun, New moon, badly associated Mercury, Mars, Saturn, Rahu and Ketu.

Moon is full from the 10th day of the bright half of the lunar month to the 5th day of the dark half of the same. He is said to be weak or new moon from the 10th day of the dark half of the lunar month to the 5th day of the bright half of the next lunar month. On other days he is said to be moderate. Mercury, by nature, is called soumya or good. And if he is in conjunction with the Sun, Saturn, Mars, Rahu or Ketu, he will be a malefic. His conjunction with beneficial planets like Full Moon, Jupiter or Venus will classify him as a benefic. Benefic means a good and malefic means an evil planet.

The influences of planets are indications of our Karmic results and by their position at birth, they indicate what the native may expect in future as the result of his previous Karma or acts.

Planetary Aspects

All planets aspect the 7th sign or the 180th degree. Jupiter aspects more powerfully in the 5th and 9th houses, Mars in the 4th and 8th houses, Saturn in the 3rd and 10th houses. Here, their influences are more effective than in the 7th house. Good aspects give beneficial results and evil aspects produce evil results. Good and evil aspects give mixed results. Planetary aspects play very important parts in the predictions of an astrologer and he must carefully mark all conjunctions, situations and aspects before venturing his predictions.

Aspects are interchanges of chemical substances at distances while conjunctions are combinations of chemicals themselves. But there are a few cases in Astrology where the aspects take the lead over conjunctions.

Planetary Relations

Among planets some are friends, others are enemies while some are classed as acquaintances and neutrals. Friendship is either permanent or temporary. Friendly planets do good; acquaintances are neutral; while enemies do evil. When planetary rays are intensified by those of another planet, he will be classed as a friend. When the rays neutralise and counteract the rays of another planet, he will be classed as a friend. When the rays neutralise and counteract the rays of another planet, both of them will be classed as enemies. When the rays are ineffective against each other, they will be termed as neutrals.

Permanent Friendship

Planets	Friends	Acquaintances	Foes
Sun	Moon, Mars, Jupiter	Mercury	Saturn, Venus
Moon	Sun, Mercury	Mars, Jupiter, Saturn, Venus	
Mars	Jupiter, Moon, Sun	Saturn, Venus	Mercury
Mercury	Sun, Venus	Mars, Jupiter, Saturn	Moon
Jupiter	Moon, Mars, Sun	Saturn	Mercury, Venus
Venus	Saturn, Mercury	Mars, Jupiter	Moon, Sun
Saturn	Venus, Mercury	Jupiter	Sun, Mars, Moon

In these classifications there are slight differences among authors. I have given the most approved theories.

Temporary Friendship

After fixing the planets in a horoscope at the time of birth, the planets occupying the 2nd, 3rd, 4th, 10th, 11th or 12th houses from any other planet become his friends. The rest are enemies. In the chart given take any planet, eg., Jupiter and see who are by position his temporary friends. Planets Moon in the 2nd, Ketu and Mars in the 11th, and Sun, Venus, Mercury and Saturn in the 12th are his friends. He has no temporary enemies as the positions of the planets are fixed here.

♓	♈ Ketu Mars	Sun, Venus, Saturn, Mercury	Jupiter
	Rasi		Birth Moon
		Rahu	

Take Rahu, planets are not found in the 2nd, 3rd, 4th, 11th and 12th houses, therefore, all these which are not there are his temporary foes. Moon is in the 10th and becomes a temporary friend. In the same way consult for other planets. There are some authors who do not apply these rules to Rahu and Ketu.

Generalisation from these principles are easy. If the two planets are friends to each other they become intimate or bosom friends. If both of them are enemies they become bitter enemies. If one is a friend and the other is an enemy, then they are called as acquaintances or neutrals.

Planetary Sexes

Jupiter, Mars and Sun are males. Venus, Rahu and Moon are females. Saturn, Mercury and Ketu are eunuchs. The influence of the planets determines the sex of the child as well as its brothers, sisters and children.

They also determine one's potency and sexual capacity.

Planetary Natures

Jupiter, Sun and Moon represent divine or sathwika and make the person mild, lover of truth, charitable, righteous, loving and philanthropic.

Venus and Mercury indicate Rajasa or imperious nature and produce men of taste, lovers of romantic enterprises, well informed in arts and sciences, fond of women, courageous and luxurious. Mars and Saturn show Thamasa or Vulgar nature and make men cheats, talebearers, quarrelsome, stubborn, lazy, cruel, vindictive, fond of sleep, indulging in mean pleasures and worthless women.

These characteristics are given to the person as the result of birth influences indicated by the planetary positions. They also largely depend upon the food he consumes, the company he keeps, the calling he pursues, and the moral training he is subjected to. It is not possible to have the planets in any one of these three states in a pure and unalloyed form. They are inclusive, but the predominating quality colours the whole life of the man and he will be classified accordingly.

Sun represents Soul or Atma or Ego. Moon represents Mind or Intellectuality. Mars represents Physical or gross nature. Mercury rules Speech, and power of eloquence. Jupiter indicates Wisdom or Vedic knowledge and Jnana, or the essence of divine wisdom. Venus shows Sexual and Worldly pleasures. Saturn represents Sorrow and Miseries.

The states or qualities represented, above will be prominent when the planets are well situated, but when they are weak, the man suffers pain or misery through these sources.

Fiery planets	Sun and Mars
Earthly planet	Mercury
Airy planet	Saturn
Divine planet	Jupiter
Watery planets	Venus and Moon

Planetary Colours

Sun	Copper
Mars	Blood Red
Moon	White
Saturn	Black
Mercury	Green
Jupiter	Bright Yellow
Venus	Mixture of all colours

But, some opine that Venus is white and he is called Sita or white.

Planetary Directions

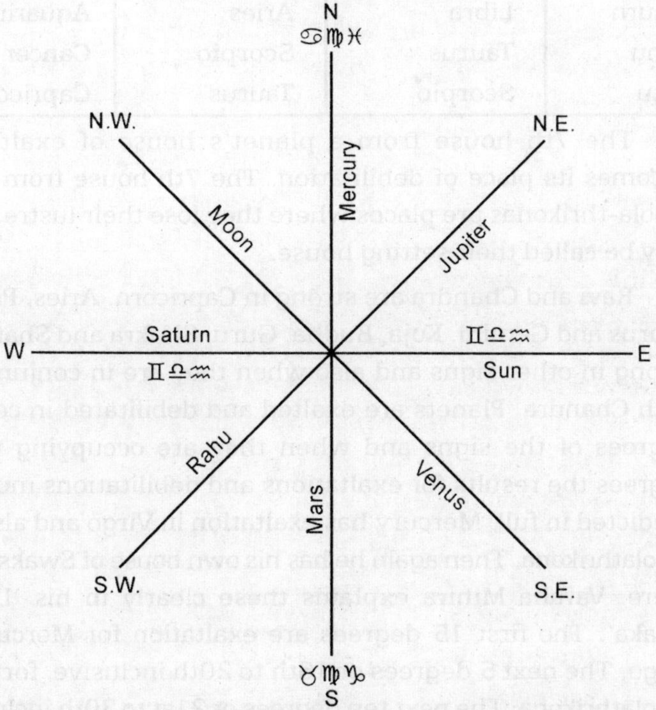

Just like planets, the Zodiacal signs also represent directions. Aries, Leo and Sagittarius represent East; Taurus, Virgo and Capricorn indicate South; Gemini, Libra and

Aquarius indicate West, and Cancer, Scorpio and Pisces represent North.

Exaltations

Planets	Houses of Exaltation	Houses of Debilitation	Moola-thrikonas
Sun	Aries	Libra	Leo
Moon	Taurus	Scorpio	Taurus
Mars	Capricorn	Cancer	Aries
Mercury	Virgo	Pisces	Virgo
Jupiter	Cancer	Capricorn	Sagittarius
Venus	Pisces	Virgo	Libra
Saturn	Libra	Aries	Aquarius
Rahu	Taurus	Scorpio	Cancer
Ketu	Scorpio	Taurus	Capricorn

The 7th house from a planet's house of exaltation becomes its place of debilitation. The 7th house from their moola-thrikonas are places where they lose their lustre. This may be called their setting house.

Ravi and Chandra are strong in Capricorn, Aries, Pisces, Taurus and Gemini. Kuja, Budha, Guru, Shukra and Shani are strong in other signs and also when they are in conjunction with Chandra. Planets are exalted and debilitated in certain degrees of the signs and when they are occupying those degrees the results for exaltations and debilitations must be predicted in full. Mercury has exaltation in Virgo and also his Moolathrikona. Then again he has his own house of Swakshetra there. Varaha Mihira explains these clearly in his 'Laghu Jataka'. The first 15 degrees are exaltation for Mercury in Virgo. The next 5 degrees or 16th to 20th inclusive, form his Moolathrikona. The next ten degrees or 21st to 30th inclusive, form his Swakshetra.

Directional Strength

Birth or Lagna represents East and Jupiter and Mercury are powerful there.

10th house indicates South and Mars and Sun are strong there.

7th house declares West and Saturn is powerful there.

4th house shows North, and Venus and Moon are auspicious there.

Planetary Movements

The sun takes one month to transit each sign. Moon completes his revolution of the whole zodiac in about 27 days, or each sign in 2¼ days.

Mars transits each sign in 45 days, Mercury and Venus take roughly a month to transit each sign.

Jupiter transits each sign in one year.

Rahu and Ketu take 18 months to transit each house.

Saturn completes his revolution of the zodiac in 30 years or takes 30 months to transit each sign.

Sun and Moon have continuous and slightly modified movements due to invisible forces called Sigrocha, Mandochha and Patha.

Excepting Rahu and Ketu, the rest of the planets viz. Mars, Mercury, Jupiter, Venus and Saturn have retrogrades or Vakrams and accelerations or Athicharas. In the former case, they move slower than usual and also move backwards and in the latter case, quicker than their allotted time and forwards. The times given here are rough and do not represent the exact velocity. The sun crosses a sign sometimes in 29 days, and on other occasions in 32 days. These differences in the Sankramana or solar transit days can be easily found out and explained in the astronomical works. The Moon, sometimes crosses a sign in 2½ days and sometimes in less than 2 days. Excepting the Sun and the Moon other planets also exhibit Stambhana (fixture) in a sign which far exceeds their allotted time. This is specially illustrated in the case of Mars, as he has got a tendency to get into fixtures very often. It should never be thought that any planet will ever remain absolutely stationary.

In Stambhana, a planet moves backwards and forwards within a narrow sphere for a longer period than its usual velocity. Take an illustration. Mars remains usually in a sign for about 45 days, but in some instances, when he gets his Stambhana, he may stay there for about 200 or even as much as 250 days. This is always followed by another state called acceleration or atichara. In this state he will cross a sign in a month or 35 days.

Conjunctional Peculiarities

Planets in conjunction with the Sun excepting Rahu and Ketu, are said to be in combustion *[Astham]*. They are then utterly powerless. Planets in conjunction with the Moon are said to be in *Samagamam* indicating good strength. If Jupiter, Venus, Mercury and Saturn are with Mars, they are said to be defeated in the planetary fight or *Grahayuddha*. If a planet is within 10 degrees then the combustion is ordinary. If a planet is beyond 15 degrees of the Sun the combustion is nominal, and will not be much injurious in results.

Strength of Time

Moon, Mars and Saturn are powerful during nights.

Mercury is always powerful.

Sun, Jupiter and Venus are strong during days.

Evil planets are strong generally during the dark halves of the lunar months, while good planets are powerful during the bright halves of the lunar months.

Saturn is the weakest, next comes Mars, then comes Mercury and then Jupiter. Venus is stronger than Jupiter, next comes Moon and Sun is the strongest of the whole lot.

Rahu and Ketu are shadowy planets which give the result of the planetary influences, according to their occupations and associations. These are Thamograhas or dark planets.

Exalted planets give full results, planets in their own houses or Moolathrikonas give 3/4 good, planets in friendly houses give 1/2 good, planets in unfriendly houses give 1/4th good and planets debilitated give no good at all, but will give evil fortune. Strength of planets can be numerically measured.

Planetary States (Avasthas)

They are:

1. **Deeptha or exaltation**: Long life, successful work, good family, promising children, wealth, fame, respect and conveyances.
2. **Swastha or residence in their own houses**: Permanent happiness, sound education, good reputation, wealth, lands, children, family comforts and good position.
3. **Mudhitha or residence in friendly signs**: Good dress, fine taste, sweet scents, flowers, women, position and happiness.
4. **Santha or planets in auspicious subdivisions**: Timely strength and courage, helping relations, comfortable life, wealth and happiness.
5. **Saktha or retrograde planets**: Courage, prosperity, successful politician, reputation, wealth, good relations and happiness.

   In retrograde, good planets produce happiness and bad planets give evil and misery.
6. **Peedya or planets in the last quarter or Navamsha of the sign**: Hatred, quarrelsome relations, family dissensions, criminal prosecutions, pilfering habits, expulsion from country.
7. **Deena or planets in unfriendly houses**: Sickness meanness, mental worry, derangement in brain, social degradation or excommunication, bigoted, persecutions.
8. **Vikala or planets in combustion**: Mental disorder, orphanage, many foes, expulsion from country, public disgrace of children, wife and friends.

9. **Khala or planets in debilitation:** Constant losses, vulgar birth, troubles from unexpected sources, quarrels with parents, imprisonment, disease, misery and utter disregard for that which is noble and sacred.

10. **Bheeta or acceleration:** Losses from fire, foes, kings and thieves, persecution, tortures, disgraceful life, vulgar habits, danger in foreign countries.

In ascribing these results, students must be careful. Suppose the Sun is exalted in Aries and has the conjunction of Saturn also there. The latter is debilitated. Suppose that instead of Saturn in conjunction, there is Jupiter in Aries along with the Sun. In predicting results either for the Sun or Saturn a large allowance must be made in both cases. Evil conjunctions and aspects add some vitality to misery; good conjunctions and good aspects are beneficial.

Similarly, in all the different states ascribed to the planets, conjunctional and aspecting influences will also have to be taken into consideration. In Astrology, like Medicine and Chemistry, the resultant of the different conjunctional forces has to be noted and calculated. Each substance may have a characteristic of its own; but when it joins with other substances chemically or otherwise, the resultant cannot and will not be the same as before and must be different. These differences have to be borne in mind by the astrologer.

Planetary Characteristics

Sun: Grey eyes, broad shoulders, bilious, bold, self-reliant, respectful, sensitive, romantic, short hairs, intelligent, stubborn, dignified, royal caste, fond of hot or pungent things, governs temples, churches, father, soul, copper, fame and dark red colour.

Moon: Sweet speech, charming eyes, windy and phlegmatic, intelligent, rounded, but not stout body, governs mother, germs, milk, mind, intelligence, watery surfaces, saltish tastes and white colour.

Mars: Youthful appearance, bilious, liberal, good pronunciation, small waist, capricious, bold, lover of dangers, military look, governs fire places, kitchens, engine rooms, armouries, gold, brothers, sisters, servants, lands, bitter tastes and red colour.

Mercury: Humorous and witty, mixed temperament, handsome countenance, prudent, cunning, good speech, governs all the baser metals, bed rooms, manufactories, eloquence, intelligence, knowledge, mixed tastes and green colour.

Jupiter: Fair, stout body, gold coloured eyes, meritorious, charitable, phlegmatic, governs priesthood, children, education, pearls, treasure rooms, physical health, wealth, sweet tastes and golden yellow colour.

Venus: Fine eyes, broad and light chest and shoulders, handsome, clever in enticing young and charming ladies, licentious, windy, phlegmatic, fond of women, refined taste, intelligent, governs bed rooms, marriage, wife, sexual pleasures, iron, wealth, vehicles, soul tastes and whitish colour.

Saturn: Dark, thin, tall and ugly body, stout bones, large teeth and thick hairs, windy temperament, base, cruel, vindictive, lazy, governs dilapidated places, tin, life, livelihood, death, acid tastes and inferior grains.

Rahu: Governs tanks, cultivation, rest houses and maternal grandparents.

Ketu: Governs grandparents, griefs, extravagance and final emancipation or Moksha.

Planetary Occupations

These are said to be 27 and the results given hereunder will be useful in timing events, after calculating Dashas or periods, (see Chapter 4).

1. **Bathing**: This indicates prosperity, good family and children, respect and successful career.
2. **Dressing**: Gems, wealth, influence, taste and clothes.

3. **Sweet scents**: Popular, gains in foreign countries, industrious and respectable.
4. **Preparation for worship**: Gain from lands, good conveyances and respectable.
5. **Praying**: Fond of lands, political troubles, loss of money and serious charges.
6. **Worship**: Wealth, popularity and favour among tyrants.
7. **Sacrificial preparation**: Bilious, distress and sound education.
8. **Meditation**: Wealthy, good relations, gains from lands, wins over foes and wealth.
9. **Kneeling**: Sweet speech, good conveyances and double-hearted.
10. **Going round the Altar**: Liver complaint, dysentery and criminal prosecution.
11. **Contemplation**: Political power, agreeable family and successful life.
12. **Reception of guests**: Conceit, magician, finder of hidden treasures.
13. **Dinner**: Cheat, sickly, and religious hatred.
14. **Drinking water**: Bad food and mean habits.
15. **Anger**: Hatred of mankind, egoistic.
16. **Chewing betel leaves**: High Service, sound education, great wealth and fame.
17. **Court entry**: Regular, pious, innocent and respectable.
18. **Crowning**: Glorious military life, great learning and wealth.
19. **Private consultation**: Laziness, sweet words, double-hearted.
20. **Delay**: Learned, dull, inactive and careless.
21. **Sleeping**: Sponge, passionate, sickly and brutal treatment towards family.

22. **Drinking**: Reckless, doing evil to friends, despising worthy people and courting ruin.
23. **Sweet drinks**: Healthy, good children, pretty wife, respected by relations and rich food.
24. **Acquisition of wealth**: Courteous, great gains and successful business.
25. **Taking off the Crown**: Loss of work, miserable, neglected by friends and relations.
26. **Profound sleep**: Chronic disease, political prosecutions and drinking.
27. **Sexual intercourse**: Much indulgence among women of disrepute, evil thoughts, melancholy, designing, suspicious and revengeful.

Persons should not run away with the idea that these occupations detailed here are being regularly performed by the planets themselves, these are resultants of light currents which planets produce from their occupation of certain houses from the birth and from birth to any other sign where a planet may be found at a given time.

The following is the simple method to find out the occupation of a given planet in any horoscope. Fix correctly the planets at the time of birth. Count from Aries always to the birth sign and keep the figure in one place. Then again count from the birth sign to the planet whose occupation is wanted and add this to the first figure, multiply the total by two and then again multiply the result by the planetary period whose occupation is needed. Divide this by 27 and the remainder shows the occupation of the planet.

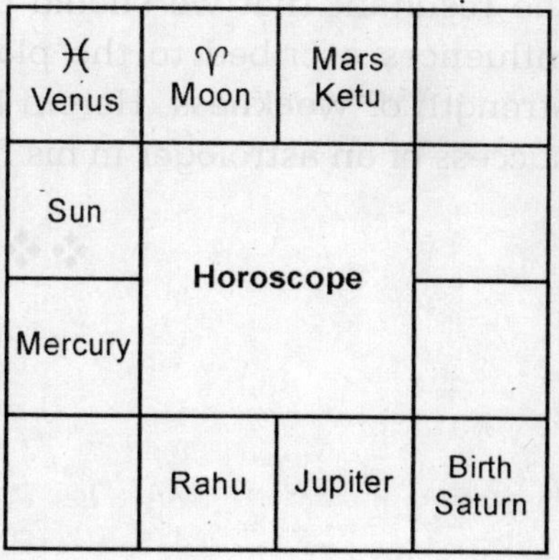

Example: A child was born at 9 p.m. on 22nd February 1863. The planets stood thus at the time. Find the Sun's occupation. Count from Aries to birth, we get 6; count again from birth to the planet Sun, we get 6, add them together we have 12, multiply this by 2, we get 24, again multiply this by the planetary period of the Sun, viz., 6 years, we have 24 x 6 = 144, divide the total by 27, we have a remainder of 9 and the occupation of the Sun in this horoscope is the 9th or kneeling and when this period comes as the result of his occupation, the Sun will give sweet, good conveyances and duplicity in character.

Take Mars and find out his occupation. Counting from Aries to birth, we get 6, from birth to the planet Mars, we get 9, adding these two we get 15, multiply this by 2, we have 30, again multiply this by 7 the period of Mars, we get 210, divide this total by 27 we get a reminder of 21.

Mars therefore is in the 21st occupation of Sleeping. When the period of Mars comes, he will give the results ascribed to him in the 21st occupation. Calculate similarly for all other planets. Astrological influences are many and various. It is the resultant that we should predict and not the separate influences ascribed to the planets in all their sources of strength or weakness. Herein lies the skill, judgement and success of an astrologer in his future predictions.

❖❖❖

CHAPTER - 3

CASTING THE HOROSCOPE

General Observations

I am giving here a general method of casting horoscopes on the basis of reliable almanacs. For detailed principles the reader is referred to Hindu Predictive Astrology by B.V. Raman.

The horoscopic chart is generally written as a square or a circle. In a circle or square the starting point may be anywhere, but to avoid mistakes I shall observe the following calculation only. The earth turns on its own axis and thus exposes always some portion of its surface to the solar influence. Lagna seems to be this surface of the earth whose distance we want to measure from the rising sign of the Sun.

As the whole earth makes one revolution in a day on its axis, all the Zodiacal signs seem to be regularly exposed to the solar influences in invariable manner, but the earth itself is not a perfect globe and being egg-shaped, sometimes we have certain signs exposed to a greater extent than others and this accounts for the short and long days and nights and differences in the time allotted to the different Zodiacal houses in different countries. Latitude and Longitude have also to be considered. The different kinds of the figures used in different parts of the world are given here for ready reference so that the student, when he looks at a horoscope may not get confused.

Pisces	Aries	Taurus	Gemini
Aquarius	No. I ZODIAC		Cancer
Capricorn			Leo
Sagittarius	Scorpio	Libra	Virgo

No. I gives the figure generally used in the Deccan and Southern India.

No. II is used in the Eastern and North-eastern parts of India.

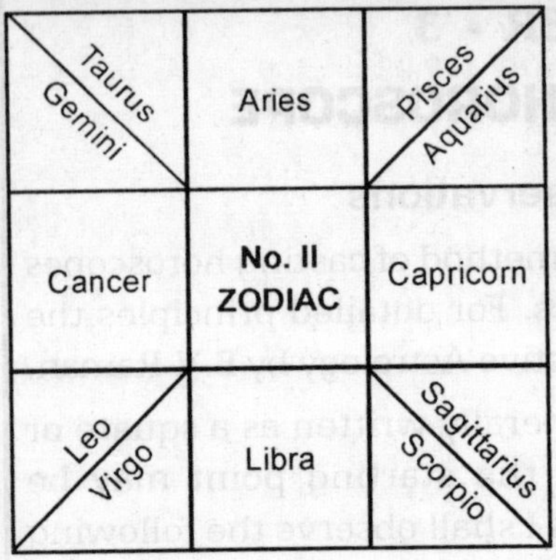

No. II

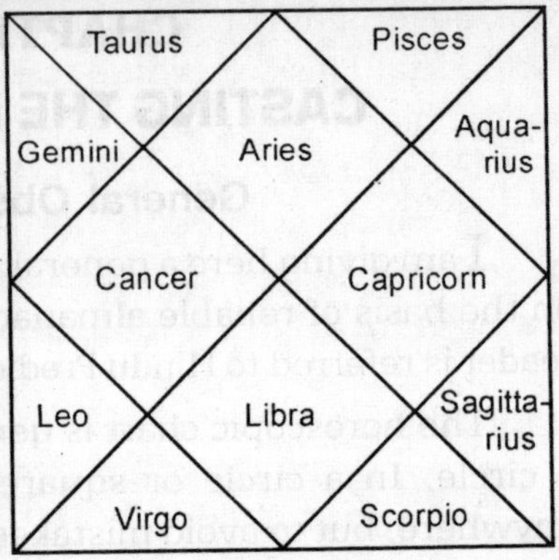

No. III

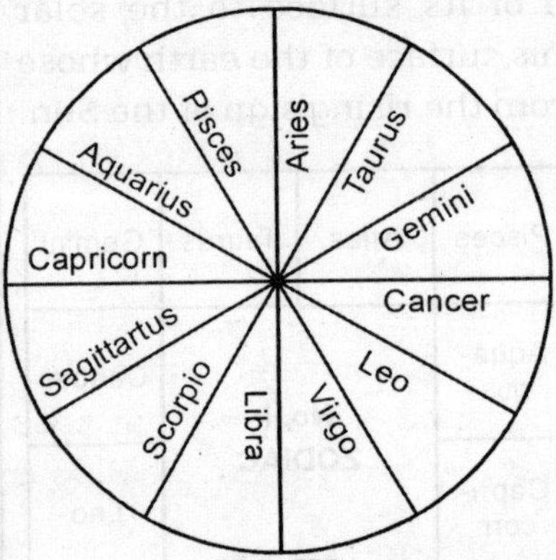

No. IV

No. III is used in the west of India and also by some of the European nations and No. IV is also used by the Indian and Continental Nations.

In all these cases excepting in No. I, we have to count from right to the left, whereas in the first we count them from left to right.

Week Days or Varas

The Maharishis give reasons for naming the week days which are thoroughly convincing. When the Sun rose, the first day in creation began and he was given Hora or influence and authority on time for 2 ghatikas on the first day and it was called Adivara (Sunday) or the first day in creation. Then came Shukra, Budha, Chandra, Manda, Guru and Kuja, respectively, and each of these governed one hora or 2 ghatikas. Then the 8th hora commenced and was governed by Ravi, the 9th by Shukra, the 10th by Budha and so on. After 14 hours, the 15th hora was again governed by Ravi and the 21st was governed by Kuja. The 22nd hora or hour was governed by the Sun, the 23rd by Shukra, and the 24th by Budha. This completed one full day or 24 horas. Therefore on the morning of the next day at sunrise, the Hora of Chandra began and it was called Soma or Chandra. Vara (Monday) after going regularly through all the horas as on the 2nd day it is found that the first hora on the 3rd day at sunrise was governed by Kuja and hence the 3rd weekday is named Bhouma, Kuja or Mangalavara (Tuesday). On the 4th day at sunrise, the hora of Budha begins and it is named Bhudhavara (Wednesday), after him on the 5th day at sunrise, the first hora was governed by Guru, and the day is called Guruvara (Thursday) after the planet. On the 6th day at sunrise, Shukra hora commences and it is called Bhrigu or Shukravara (Friday). On the 7th day at sunrise, the first hora was ruled by Shani and it goes after him, viz., Shanivara (Saturday), on the 8th day again at sunrise the first hora was governed by Ravi and on the 9th day Chandra and so forth.

No other literature seems to offer such easy and comprehensible explanation for naming the weekdays as the Hindus have done and these processes refer to times long before the dawn of modern civilisation. All the nations seem to have borrowed their names for the weekdays from the Hindus.

Conversion of Time

A day is divided into 60 equal divisions called Ghatikas, therefore an English hour = 2½ Ghatis. A Ghatika is again divided into 60 Vighatikas and therefore 2½ Vighatikas make an English minute. For ordinary calculations this is enough. I shall here state some divisions of time which the ancient Hindu Maharishis made and the influences of the minuteness of Time as discovered by them. Facts will speak for themselves. English Time (24 hours for a day, 60 minutes for an hour, 60 seconds for a minute) exhausts their idea of minute divisions of time and we get therefore for a day, $24 \times 60 \times 60 = 86{,}400$ seconds. Beyond seconds they have no conception of names for still minuter divisions of time. Let us see what the Hindus say about time.

A day is comprised of 60 ghatikas. Each ghatika has 60 vighatikas. Each vighatika has 60 liptas, each lipta has 60 viliptas, each vilipta has 60 paras and each para has 60 tatparas. One day therefore contains 46,656,000,000 tatparas. While the Western astronomers and mathematicians divide one day into 86,400 seconds or five digits, the Hindu Siddhantees have gone into 11 figures (digits), the mathematical readers will see the force of this statement and the keenness of intellects which can go so minutely into the divisions of time. When a second is the minutest division of Western astronomy, this second has been divided into 540,000 divisions called Tatparas by the ancient Hindu astronomers.

A day means one rotation of the Earth on its own axis and therefore, the exposure of the whole of its surface to the solar influence. Thus the 12 signs into which the Earth is marked are regularly exposed to the Sun one after another everyday. And the 12 solar months are named after the Zodiacal signs which are first exposed to the Sun during the particular period at sunrise. We have Aries ascending in the first month, that is Aries is first exposed to solar influence. Then Taurus, then Gemini, then Cancer and so on.

For the sake of convenience they have divided Aries into 30 equal divisions, called degrees and on the first day of Aries we see the sunrise in the 1st degree of it, on the 2nd day in the 2nd degree, on the 3rd day in the 3rd degree and so on, until on the 30th day of the solar month of the Aries, we have the sunrise almost at the end of Aries or in its 30th degree. Next day we see the sunrise not in Aries, but in the 1st degree of Taurus. Thus on the 60th day we see the sunrise in the 30th degree of Taurus and at the end of 365 days composing the solar year we see the sunrise in the 30th degree of Pisces or the last degree of the Zodiac. The Sun therefore, gains, as it were, a degree everyday in the Zodiac. It would be out of place to go into further details in a small book of this nature. Every day, therefore, we have the following periods of time assigned to the Zodiacal signs which go once round in a day and which are regularly exposed to solar influences during the times. The Latitude and Meridian have direct bearing in determining these divisions of time. The following table gives the different times allotted roughly for the Deccan. For careful calculations the Akshamshas have to be consulted. (Latitudes)

One day is composed of the following durations of signs at the Equator:—

Zodiacal Signs	Ghatikas	Vighatikas	Hrs.	Mts.
Aries — Mesha	4	00	1	36
Taurus — Vrishabha	4	30	1	48
Gemini — Mithuna	5	15	2	06
Cancer — Kataka	5	30	2	12
Leo—Simha	5	30	2	12
Virgo—Kanya	5	15	2	06
Libra—Thula	5	15	2	06
Scorpio—Vrischika	5	30	2	12
Sagittarius—Dhanus	5	30	2	12
Capricorn—Makara	5	15	2	06
Aquarius—Kumbha	4	30	1	48
Pisces—Meena	4	00	1	36
Total - 12 Signs	60 Ghatikas		24 Hours	

This table is applicable only to Deccan in a general manner.

These tables cannot be correct for any part of the world. If the earth is egg-shaped or oval then the extent of the signs must vary in each country according to its distance from the equator and the latitude and the longitude of the place itself. These tables which check the different measurements of the signs in different countries are called "Deshanthara Samskaras" in astronomy and every student who wishes to be correct must be familiar with the principles of correctly calculating the positions of the planets and the extent of the Zodiac which constitutes any sign particularly.

Horoscope Casting

The following is reproduced from Hindu predictive Astrology by B.V. Raman:

Find out the date of birth in the almanac for the particular year and write on a sheet of paper all the details given for that day. In most of the almanacs the positions of the planets are given in Nakshatra padas or quarters and by merely copying them one would be able to mark the Rasi (Zodiacal) and Navamsha (one-ninth division) diagrams.

Ascertain the exact moment of birth and sunrise. If the time is in English hours, convert it into ghaties (2½ ghaties make one hour, 24 minutes make one ghati and 24 seconds make one lipti). If the birth has occurred after midnight it must be taken as belonging to the previous day as among the Hindus, a day is reckoned from sunrise to sunrise. Ascertain how many hours after sunrise the birth has occurred and convert this into ghaties.

In the almanac, if there are any planets marked on the day of birth and if the ghaties given against each or any of them are below the time of birth, reproduce them as they are, otherwise, trace back and find out the positions of planets nearest to the date of birth. For the Moon, some calculations are necessary. Find out the constellation on the day of birth which can be readily seen in the almanac and note down its duration. If it be the one that ends on the same day, then add to this duration the number of ghaties and vighaties obtained by subtracting from 60, the extent of the preceding asterism on the previous day. The sum represents the entire duration of the constellation in question.

One fourth of this gives the duration of a quarter or pada. Add birth time to the duration of the constellation on the previous day. This gives how much of time has elapsed in the constellation at the time of birth. Dividing this by the duration of each quarter, we get the particular quarter of the constellation which the Moon is on.

In case the Constellation be the one that ends on the next day, then find the duration of the asterism on the day of birth and that on the next day must be obtained thus:

The sunrise on the day of the following illustrative horoscope is approximately at 5.35 a.m. and the birth has taken place at 5.35 p.m. Deducting sunrise from birth time (5.35 p.m. = 17 hours 35 minutes) we get 12 hours. This converted into ghaties at 2½ ghaties per one hour gives 30 ghaties as the time of birth the constellation Rohini ruled for 21-50 ghaties. Subtract from 60 ghaties, the number of ghaties and vighaties at which the Moon left the previous constellation. Add to this, the number of ghaties and vighaties when the constellation terminates the next day. The total duration of the constellation is obtained. Subtract from the time of birth (in ghaties) the time when the Moon left the previous asterism. The time elapsed from the beginning of the constellation to the moment of the birth is obtained. Now it will be easy to find in what quarter the Moon is placed.

The following illustration enables the student to grasp the principles enumerated above easily.

Illustration: Born 8th August 1912 A.D. at 5.35 p.m. Long 78 E., Latitude 10 N.

On 8-8-1912		**On 9-8-1912**
Duration of the day =	Gh. 60-00	Extent of Mrighasira =
Extent of Rohini	21-59	Gh. 19-15
Extent of Mrigasira	38-1	

Extent of Mrigasira =

On 8-8-1912

Total duration of Mrigasira =		38-1
		19-15
		57-16

Dividing this by 4, we get that each quarter lasts for

$$\frac{57-16}{4} = \text{Gh. } 14\text{-}19$$

Again, Birth Time	Gh.	30-00
Duration of Rohini	Gh.	21-59
Time elapsed in Mrigashira	Gh.	8-1

Since the balance is less than ghaties 14-19 the first quarter of Mrigasira rules at birth, i.e., the Moon occupies the first quarter of Mrighasira. Tracing back, the positions of other planets are obtained thus:

Sun in the	II	quarter of	Ashlesha
Moon	I	-do-	Mrigasira
Mars	III	-do-	Pubba
Mercury	II	-do-	Makha (Retrogression)
Jupiter	II	-do-	Jyeshta
Venus	I	-do-	Makha
Saturn	I	-do-	Rohini
Rahu	III	-do-	Revati
Ketu	I	-do-	Chitra

Take the Sun. He is in the II quarter of Ashlesha Count from the constellation Aswini up to the constellation of the planet. It is 8. Convert this into padas or quarters, (one quarter is equal to $3\frac{1}{3}$ degrees of ecliptic arc), 8x4 = 32.

Add two quarters already passed by the planet in Aslesha. 32 + 2 = 34. Since 9 padas make one Rashi, divide this by 9, 34/ 9 = 3. The remainder is 7. That is, the Sun has passed three signs from Aries and is in the fourth sign, namely, Cancer.

Similarly fix all the other planets in their respective signs.

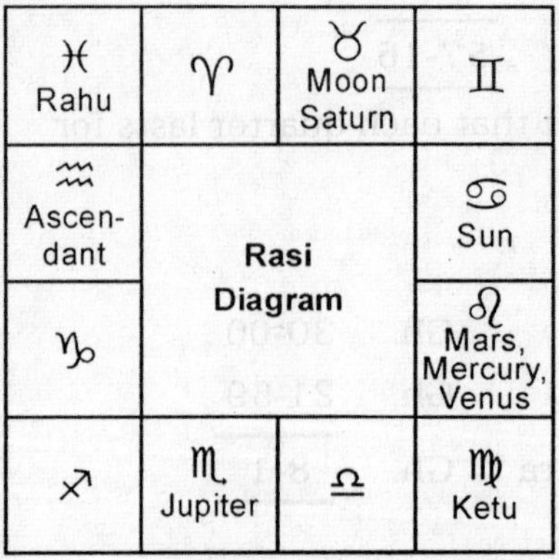

Lagna (Ascendant)

The process next to that of fixing the planets lies in the correct determination of Lagna or the ascendant.

The duration of the signs varies in accordance with the degree of the latitude of the place.

The degree and the sign in which the Sun rises will be the ascendant at that particular time. The solar date of birth is readily found out in the almanac. In the illustration given, the solar date is the 24th of Cancer. The rising sign in that month will be Cancer itself. But the Sun rises in it on the first day in the first degree of Cancer. The person was born on the 24th evening and therefore the Sun has passed 23 degrees of Cancer and rose on that morning in the 24th degree.

Therefore, the Sun on the day of birth was in Cancer 24 degrees. Time of birth is 30 ghaties. Cancer extends for 5-30 ghaties. Therefore each degree requires 5-30 × 60/30 = 11 vighaties to rise. Therefore the Sun has gained 23 × 11 = 253 vighaties or 4 ghaties and 13 vighaties.

	Ghaties
Duration of Cancer	5 - 30
Ghaties gained by the Sun	4 - 13
Ghaties remaining to be covered by the Sun	1 - 17
Leo	5 - 30
Virgo	5 - 15
Libra	5 - 15
Scorpio	5 - 30
Sagittarius	5 - 30
Total	28 - 17

Birth has taken place at 30 ghaties and since Sagittarius closes at 28-17 after sunrise, the Ascendant is Capricorn, i.e. 1 ghati and 43 vighaties have elapsed in Capricorn.

Casting the Planetary Chart "Indian Ephemeris"

The latest Indian Ephemeris by Lahiri or the Rashtreeya Panchanga of the Government of India give the Planetary Longitudes of all the planets at 5.30 a.m. Indian Standard Time. These longitudes are astronomically accurate and are universally true too. Thus the latest method of casting the Horoscope is according to the modern ephemeris – Indian or Foreign.

Calculation of planetary positions for a given moment is self-evident. Get familiarised with the various contents of the 'Indian Ephemeris' currently popular. The planetary longitudes for the day at 5.30 a.m. corresponding to the 0.00 hour of G.M.T. are recorded. Daily average motion of the planets are given there. The difference between two successive days concerned gives the motion of the planet for the day. Calculate the Elapsed Time of the moment from the Ephemeris time (5.30 a.m.) Calculate the proportional motion of the planets for the elapsed time and add it to its longitude of the day. This gives the longitude of the planet for the required moment. It is notified that no considerable difference would occur if the Local Mean Time of the place is not taken instead of the Indian Standard Time. Mathematical accuracy is everybody's desire. Approximations are not accuracies.

General procedure for the computation of the Ascendant for a given moment is detailed in another important book by the same author — Lahiri, namely 'Table of Ascendants'. Practice under guidance of an adept is preferable. Ascendant of the given moment and the correct longitudes of the planets are the two most basically important aspects of Astrological Predictions. Sidhanta - the mathematical part and phala - the predictive part, pivot round the accuracy of the Ascendant and the planetary longitudes of the moment. Some worked examples shall illustrate the present procedure step by step.

Note: Refer pages 3, 4, 5 and 6 of Indian Ephemeris by Lahiri for explanation and details of longitudes sidereal time, Thithi, Nakshatra, Prefixes and Suffixes used in it, dates of Indian National Calendar; symbols used for signs and planets and circular distances and measures of time, as also different eras in vogue locally, are explained. A close study is essential before making use of it. Proportional logarithms for quicker calculations with many useful tables are provided.

❖❖❖

CHAPTER - 4

PLANETARY PERIODS AND SUB-PERIODS OR DASHAS AND BHUKTHIES

Determine the constellation in which the Moon is placed at the time of birth and ascribe the planetary periods as given below:

This system is known as Udu Dasha from Udu meaning a Nakshatra or constellation. It is also styled Vimshottari or 120 years. The total of all the Dashas will come up to 120 years system. There are other systems recommended in the Astrological works, but as they involve some calculations which may be difficult for beginners, I have given the simplest system possible. Ashtottari or 108 years system, prevails generally in Northern India. The Dashas and Antardashas given in the Brihat Jataka, based on the position and strength of the planets in the kendras, panaparas and apoklimas are elaborately explained by me in my notes in the English Translation of Brihat Jataka to which I refer my readers for fuller details.

The First Dasha begins with Krittika.

Sun's Dasha or period 6 years. Krittika—3, Uttara phalguni — 12, Uttarashada—21.

Moon's period 10 years. Rohini—4, Hasta—13, Shravana—22.

Mars' period 7 years. Mrigasira—5, Chitra—14, Dhanishta— 23.

Rahu's period 18 years. Arudra—6, Swati—15, Satabisha—24.

Jupiter's period 16 years. Punarvasu—7, Visakha—16, Poorvabhadra—25.

Saturn's period 19 years, Pushya—8, Anuradha—17, Uttarabhadra— 26.

Mercury's period 17 years. Aslesha—9, Jyeshta— 18, Revati—27.

Ketu's period 7 years. Makha—10, Moola—19, Ashwini—1.

Venus' period 20 years. Poorvaphalguni—11, Poorvashada—20, Bharani—2.

The numeral figures marked against the constellations indicate the number from Aswini or the first star.

Find out the ascending constellation at the time of birth and fix the planetary period by referring to this table. As permanent laws are subjected to local or temporary laws, so also general influences of the planets are subjected to the particular influences of the planetary periods. The total number of years of these periods gives us 120 years, generally supposed to be the term of man's life.

The position of the Moon at birth determines the ruling period. And the next Dashas succeed in the order given above. Take an example: The Moon is in the first quarter of Bharani. Therefore Venus rules the native at birth. If the Moon were in the very beginning of Bharani, Venus would control this native for the full period of 20 years assigned to him. But suppose 10 ghaties have already passed in Bharani which means the corresponding period must be deducted out of the Dasha of Venus.

If the duration of constellation is say 60 ghaties then we may ask if 60 ghaties give 20 years, what will 10 ghaties give?

60 : 20 :: 10 : required number of years.

$\frac{20 \times 10}{60}$ years 3—4—0, $\left(3\frac{1}{3}\text{ years}\right)$

	Years	Months	Days
Total Dasha of Venus	20	0	0
Expired period (lapsed)	3	4	0
Balance of the Dasha at Birth	16	8	0

Apart from the good and bad that is given generally by the planetary combinations, at the time of birth, we have also to take into consideration the present movement of the heavenly luminaries and see how these two sets of influences act or react on each other. If a superior is good and his subordinate is bad, then the applicant finds some delay at least, in the disposal of his papers and vice versa. If both are good, he will have immediate success and if both are bad he will be unsuccessful. It is very essential, therefore, that these rules must be carefully remembered. The planets shed their influences. These different types of the planets act and react upon each other. Results are produced from such actions and reactions, some rays are intensified, some counteract each other and some remain neutral.

Planets go on revolving round each other in endless varieties and each planetary period has sub-periods and other minor divisions. Principally we have Dasha or chief period, where the planet has a general control, Vidasha or Antardasha or sub-period. Antarantaradasha or minor period, Sookshmadasha or very minute period and pranadasha or minutest period.

Take the period of Ravi. First the planets revolve round each other in the following order given already in treating of the constellations and planetary periods Ravi, Chandra, Kuja, Rahu, Guru, Shani, Buddha, Ketu and Shukra. In every period we have to observe the same order of planets in all these sub and other minor periods. Take the period of Ravi, it is 6 years. Ravi now has a certain portion in the general period of life fixed for man, viz, 120 years, according to the Udu Dasha, and this proportion he holds constantly in all periods, and their divisions, however minute they may be. As 120 is to 6 years (the Principal Period of Ravi), so is 6 to the period of Ravi

$$= \frac{6 \times 6}{120} \text{ year, b} = \frac{6}{20} = \frac{3}{10} \times 12 \text{ months}$$

$$\frac{36}{10} = 3 \text{ months} \quad \frac{6}{10} \times 30 \text{ days} = 18 \text{ days.}$$

Thus in Ravi's principal period, Ravi's sub-period is 3 months and 18 days.

For Chandra we have 120 : 10 :: 6

$\frac{60}{120}$ = years = 6 months.

But there is another method very easily remembered and I shall state that here for ready reference. Multiply the number of the principal period of the planet by the number of the years of the principal period of the planet whose sub-period is required, and multiply the last figure only by 3 and keep it as days, and the first one or two figures as the case may be, as months only. Thus for Ravi in Ravi we have 6 × 6 = 36, here multiply the last figure 6 by 3 we have 18 days, and the first figure is 3 months.

Now take Chandra in Ravi. Ravi = 6 × 10 = 60, the last is a zero and therefore gives us no value in days when multiplied by 3 and the first is 6 months.

Take Kuja in Ravi = 7 × 6 = 42, we get 4 months and 6 days.

Take Rahu in Ravi =18 × 6= 108, we have 10 months and 18 days, in the same way calculate for all other planets.

I have given a table at the end of this chapter for ready reference.

It is seen that Ravi's sub-period is 3 months and 24 days. I have shown already that the planets bear the same proportion invariable in all periods, sub-periods and other divisions as they have in the general period of 120 years.

If in 120 years, Ravi gets 6 years, how much does he get in

$3\frac{18}{30}$ months. Therefore $\frac{108}{120} \times 6 = 5\frac{8}{20}$ days

This is the period of Ravi's Antardarsha in Ravi's Vidasha in Ravi's Dasha.

Again 120 : 6 :: 5 $\frac{2}{5}$:? The answer = $\frac{6\times27}{120\times5}$

= $\frac{27}{100}$ days for Ravi. This is Ravi's Antarantardasha.

To get Sookshma Dasha we have again to follow the same process.

$$120: \frac{27}{100} :: 6 = \frac{27}{100} \times \frac{6}{120} = \frac{27\times6}{12000}$$

$$\frac{27}{2000} \times 24 \times 60 \text{ minutes} = \frac{3\times9\times4\div6}{2000}$$

$$= 60 = 3 \times 3 \times 3 = 19 \text{ minutes and } 26\frac{2}{5} \text{ seconds.}$$

To get the Prana Dasha, the Sookshma result will again have to be similarly dealt with. In the same way it must be consulted for other planets to get the minutest periods of these influences in their revolutions in space.

Table of Planetary Periods and Sub-periods

Period	Sub-period	Months	Days	Period	Sub-period	Months	Days	Remarks
Ravi	Ravi	3	18	Chan-dra	Chandra	10	–	Ravi's period is 6 years Chandra's is 10 years
	Chandra	6	00		Kuja	7	–	
	Kuja	4	6		Rahu	18	–	
	Rahu	10	24		Guru	16	–	
	Guru	9	18		Shani	19	–	
	Shani	11	12		Budha	7	–	
	Budha	10	06		Ketu	7	–	
	Ketu	4	06		Shukra	20	–	
	Shukra	12	00		Ravi	6	–	
Kuja	Kuja	4	27	Rahu	Rahu	32	12	Kuja's is 7 years, Rahu's is 18 years
	Rahu	12	18		Guru	28	24	
	Guru	11	06		Shani	34	06	
	Shani	13	09		Budha	30	18	
	Budha	11	27		Ketu	12	18	
	Ketu	4	27		Shukra	36	00	
	Shukra	14	00		Ravi	10	24	
	Ravi	4	06		Chandra	18	00	
	Chandra	7	00		Kuja	12	18	
Guru	Guru	25	18	Shani	Shani	36	03	Guru's is 16 years, Shani's is 19 years
	Shani	30	12		Budha	32	09	
	Budha	27	06		Ketu	13	09	
	Ketu	11	06		Shukra	38	00	
	Shukra	32	00		Ravi	11	12	
	Ravi	9	18		Chandra	19	00	
	Chandra	16	00		Kuja	13	09	
	Kuja	11	06		Rahu	34	16	
	Rahu	28	24		Guru	30	12	
Budha	Budha	28	27	Ketu	Ketu	4	27	Budha's is 17 years, Ketu's is 7 years
	Ketu	11	27		Shukra	14	00	
	Shukra	34	00		Ravi	4	06	
	Ravi	10	06		Chandra	7	00	
	Chandra	17	00		Kuja	4	27	
	Kuja	11	27		Rahu	12	18	
	Rahu	30	18		Guru	11	06	
	Guru	27	06		Shani	13	09	
	Shani	32	09		Budha	11	27	

Shukra's period is 20 years

Shukra - Shukra - 40 Months
Shukra - Ravi - 12 Months
Shukra - Chandra - 20 Months
Shukra - Kuja - 14 Months
Shukra - Rahu - 36 Months
Shukra - Guru - 32 Months
Shukra - Shani - 38 Months
Shukra - Budha - 34 Months
Shukra - Ketu - 14 Months

CHAPTER - 5

ZODIACAL DIVISIONS

HORA

When a sign is divided into two equal parts, each part is called a *Hora.* In odd signs the 1st and 2nd Horas are ruled by the Sun and the Moon respectively. In even signs the first is governed by the Moon and the second by the Sun. A Hora gets 15 degrees.

DREKKANA

When a sign is divided into three equal parts, each part is called a Drekkana. The lord of the first drekkana is the lord of the sign itself. The lord of the second drekkana is the lord of the 5th sign from it; and the lord of the third drekkana is the lord of the 9th sign from the first.

Example 1: Take Aries. Divide it into three equal parts. First part is governed by the lord of the sign Mars. Second part is ruled by the lord of the 5th sign Leo or the Sun. Third part is ruled by the lord of the 9th sign Sagittarius or Jupiter.

Example 2: Take Virgo. First part is ruled by Mercury, lord of the house. Second part by Saturn, lord of the 5th sign Capricorn. Third part is ruled by Venus lord of the 9th house Taurus. Consider others in the same way. Each drekkana gets 10 degrees.

NAVAMSHA

When a sign is divided into 9 equal parts, each is called a Navamsha. Here the lords commence from Aries and continue their rounds regularly without any break. Therefore a clear explanation is necessary as the beginners are liable to be confused.

Take Aries. Divide it into nine equal parts. First Navamsha is governed by its lord Mars, 2nd is governed by the lord of the 2nd Taurus, viz., Venus; 3rd Navamsha is governed by the lord of the 3rd sign Gemini, viz., Mercury, and so on the last Navamsha is governed by the lord of the 9th house Sagittarius, viz., Jupiter. After Aries, we come next to Taurus, and here, the 1st Navamsha, instead of being governed by its lord, is governed by the lord of the 10th from Aries, where we have left off for counting from Aries and from where we must commence for Taurus, and the lord of the 10th house Capricorn is Saturn. The 2nd Navamsha of Taurus is governed by the lord of the next house Aquarius and he is Saturn, the third Navamsha of Taurus is Pisces and its lord Jupiter governs it and so the 9th Navamsha of Taurus is Virgo and its lord is Mercury so that the 1st Navamsha of the next sign Gemini is Libra and Venus is its lord, the 2nd Navamsha of Gemini is Scorpio and Mars is its lord, the 9th Navamsha of Gemini is Gemini itself and Mercury governs it.

For Cancer the 1st Navamsha is Cancer and Moon is its lord, the 9th Navamsha is Pisces and Jupiter is its lord.

For Leo, we commence from Aries again. Thus the result of these calculations is, for Aries, Leo and Sagittarius count regularly the navamsha from Aries; for Taurus, Virgo and Capricorn count from Capricorn, for Gemini, Libra and Aquarius count from Libra, and for Cancer, Scorpio and Pisces count from Cancer. The lords of the houses are the lords of the Navamshas. Each Navamsha gets 2½ degrees.

DWADASHAMSHA

Divide a sign into twelve equal parts and each part is called a Dwadashamsha. For any sign count regularly from the sign itself. For Aries the first Dwadashamsha is Aries. Second is Taurus, and the 12th is Pisces. For Taurus, 1st is itself and 12th is Aries, and for other signs, calculate in the same way. Each Dwadashamsha gets 2½ degrees.

TRIMSHAMSHA

When a sign is divided into thirty equal parts, each is called a Trimshamsha. In odd signs first 5 parts are governed by Mars, the next five parts by Saturn, the next 8 parts by

Jupiter, the next 7 parts by Mercury and the last 5 parts by Venus.

In even signs the reverse is the case, thus the first 5 parts are ruled by Venus, next 7 parts by Mercury, next 8 parts by Jupiter, next 5 parts by Saturn and the last 5 parts by Mars.

In Odd signs we have:

Mars		Saturn		Jupiter		Mercury		Venus		
5	+	5	+	8	+	7	+	5	=	30 parts

In Even signs:

Venus		Mercury		Jupiter		Saturn		Mars		
5	+	7	+	8	+	5	+	5	=	30 parts

There are other minute subdivisions, but it is not desirable to go so deep into those details in a small book of this nature. Each Trimshamsha gets one degree in the sign.

Lagna, Hora, Drekkana, Navamsha, Dwadashamsha and Trimshamsha are called the Shadvargas or 6 important divisions of the zodiacal signs. Planets in good Vargas are productive of favourable results. The birth sign shares a similar fate.

When a sign is divided into sixty equal divisions each of them is called a Shashtiamsha.

In even signs the order here given must be accepted, while in odd signs it must be reversed. In the even signs we go on with 1, 2, 3, 4 etc., and in odd signs we commence with 60, 59, 58, 57, 56, etc., or count in the reverse order.

In even signs the Shashtiamshas are:

(1) Ghoramsha: bad **(2)** Rakshasa: bad **(3)** Devabhaga: good **(4)** Kuberamsha: good **(5)** Rakshogana: good **(6)** Kinnera: good **(7)** Bhrashta: bad **(8)** Kulaghna: bad **(9)** Garala: bad **(10)** Agnisangha: bad **(11)** Mayamsha: bad **(12)** Prata-purisha: bad **(13)** Apampathi: good **(14)** Devangana: good **(15)** Kala: bad **(16)** Ahi: bad **(17)** Amritamsha: good **(18)** Chandramsha: good **(19)** Mriduvamsha: good **(20)** Komala: good **(21)** Padmabhaga: good **(22)** Lakshmisha:

good **(23)** Vagisha: good **(24)** Digambara: good **(25)** Davamsa: good **(26)** Indramsha: good **(27)** Kalinasha: good **(28)** Kshitiswara: good **(29)** Karmalakara: good **(30)** Mumdathmaja: bad **(31)** Mrityamsha: bad **(32)** Kala: bad **(33)** Davangi: bad **(34)** Chora: bad **(35)** Amritha: good **(36)** Garala: bad **(37)** Agnisangha: bad **(38)** Mayamsha: bad **(39)** Paripurna: good **(40)** Vishapradagdha: bad **(41)** Kalinasha: good **(42)** Mookhya: good **(43)** Vamshakshaya: bad **(44)** Ootpatha: bad **(45)** Kalapura: bad **(46)** Soumya: good **(47)** Mridwamsha: good **(48)** Sushithala: good **(49)** Dounstrakarala: bad **(50)** Indumukha: good **(51)** Pravina: good **(52)** Kalagni: bad **(53)** Dandayudha: bad **(54)** Niramalamsha: good **(55)** Subha: good **(56)** Ashubha: bad **(57)** Athithalumsha: bad **(58)** Sudhapayodhi: good **(59)** Dyumani: good **(60)** Indurakha: good.

Planets have 10 Vargas and they are:

(1) Powerful planets **(2)** exalted planets **(3)** planets in moolathrikonas **(4)** planets in their own houses **(5)** planets in quadrants **(6)** planets in good amshas **(7)** planets in friendly houses **(8)** planets in trines **(9)** planets in their own navamshas and **(10)** planets in their adhimitramshas.

A Varga in Sanskrit means a division. This may be Shubha (good) or Ashubha (evil).

When a planet has 3 vargas it will be Uttamamsha.

When a planet has 4 vargas it is Gopuramsha.

When it has 5 vargas it is Simhasanamsha.

When it has 2 vargas it is called Parijathamsha.

When it has 6 vargas it is called Parvathamsha.

When it has 7 vargas it is Devalokamsha.

When it has 8 vargas it is Kunkumamsha.

When it has 9 vargas it is Iravatamsha.

When it has 10 vargas it is Visheshakamsha.

When a planet occupies a certain number of vargas or good divisions of the Zodiacal sign, it gets into a favourable state and produces some good results. A short description is given here.

In Iravatamsha the planet makes a man an emperor, immensely wealthy and very famous.

In Devalokamsha, very liberal, a Maharaja and famous.

In Parvathamsha, many maternal uncles, well educated and influential.

In Simhasanamsha, well praised for his merits a great Raja or statesman; a rich zamindar or land holder.

In Uttamamsha, blessed with all comforts.

In Parijatamsha, wealthy.

❖❖❖

CHAPTER - 6

PECULIARITIES OF SIGNS, ZODIACAL DIVISIONS ETC.

ORGANS OF KALAPURUSHA

Time personified in a vedantic sense is called Kalapurusha and the Zodiacal signs govern the following organs of Kalapurusha indicating influences on the special organs sketched below:

1. Aries—head—Sira
2. Taurus—face—Mukha
3. Gemini—chest—Uru
4. Cancer—heart—Hrit
5. Leo—belly—Kroda
6. Virgo—lions—Vasobhrita
7. Libra—abdomen—Vasti
8. Scorpio—sexual organs—Vyanjana
9. Sagittarius—thighs—Ooru
10. Capricorn—knees—Janu
11. Aquarius—buttocks—Jangha
12. Pisces—feet—Anghri

After finding the planets at the time of birth, look out for the different organs of the body with reference to this table and whichever organs are occupied by evil planets, predict disease or pain there according to the intensity of the influences, and whichever are aspected by good planets, say there will be less pain, and whichever organs are occupied by good planets, predict health and vigour in those organs.

PECULIARITIES OF THE SIGNS

Sings are divided into movable, fixed and common or Chara, Sthira and Dwiswabhava.

Movable signs are: Aries and its quadrants or Cancer, Libra and Capricorn.

Fixed signs are: Taurus, Leo, Scorpio and Aquarius.

Common signs are: Gemini, Virgo, Sagittarius and Pisces.

Masculine and cruel signs are: Aries, Gemini and other odd signs.

Feminine and mild signs are: Taurus, Cancer and other even signs.

Nocturnal signs are: Aries, Taurus, Gemini, Cancer, Capricorn; these with the exception of Gemini are also called Prushtodaya (rising by hinder part).

Diurnal signs are: Leo, Libra, Virgo, Scorpio, Aquarius; these with Gemini form Sirshodaya (rising by head). Pisces forms a combination of the above two and is called Ubhayodaya (rising by head and hinder part).

Quadrants or Kendras are: 1st, 4th, 7th and 10th houses from birth or Lagna. Here good planets give beneficial influences. Evil planets are not so effective in producing good. Sun and Mars in the 10th are very powerful and Saturn in the 7th is good.

Trines or Trikonas are: 1st, 5th and 9th houses. Here also good planets give much good. First is already included in the Kendra, therefore, only 5th and 9th have to be specifically considered as Trikonas.

Panaparas or next house to quadrants are: 2nd, 5th, 8th and 11th houses. Fifth is a Trikona.

Apoklimas or next house to the above are: 3rd, 6th and 9th and 12th houses.

Ninth is a Trikona and must be excluded.

Upachayas or improving houses: 3rd, 9th, 10th and 11th houses.

INDICATIONS OF SIGNS

1. **Aries**: *Resembles a ram*—indicates head and governs shrubs, inferior jungles, caves, hills, mineral tracts and fiery places.
2. **Taurus**: *A bull-neck*—forest, mountains, cattle—sheds, cultivated fields.
3. **Gemini**: *A man with a club and a woman holding a lute facing each other*—shoulders, musicians, dancing women, carpenters, places of sexual intercourse, gambling house and pleasure walks.
4. **Cancer**: *A crab*—chest, watery places, sand banks, holy places and angelic sites.

5. **Leo**: *A lion*—heart, forests, caves, hunting places, inaccessible peaks and rocks.
6. **Virgo**: *A virgin with a lamp in hand seated in a boat on water*—stomach, arts, green meadows, women, industries and places of enjoyment.
7. **Libra**: *A man seated in a thoroughfare with articles of sale and a balance in hand*—navel, loins, abdomen, commercial streets, roads, cities, large towns, companies of merchants or dealers and high places of cultivation.
8. **Scorpio**: *A scorpion in an underground hole*—sexual organs and rectum, natural crevices, dark retreats, molehills, insects, serpents of all description and wild places.
9. **Sagittarius**: *A centaur*—things, plains, camping grounds, chariots, horses, armouries, sacrificial places, stables and weapons.
10. **Capricorn**: *Half beast and half crocodile*—knees, calves, rivers, watery places, jungles and opening in the ground.
11. **Aquarius**: *A water-bearer*—lower half of the leg, watery and marshy places, fields yielding inferior grains, places where birds congregate in large numbers, rendezvous of vulgar women, toddy shops and gambling places.
12. **Pisces**: *Two fishes with the face of the one turned towards the face of the other*—governs feet, watery places, holy shrines, places of pilgrimage, sacred rivers, oceans and large watery expanses, tanks and congress of holy men.

These indications of signs will be found to be useful in finding out places where the thieves have run away or where the lost articles may be traced or hidden. They also show the tendencies or objects governed by them.

SIGNIFICATION OF THE HOUSES

First house (Lagna): Nature, birth, maternal labour, complexion, physical features and spirit.

Second house: Wealth, power of speech, family, eyes, journeys, face, metals and gold.

Third house: Brothers, sisters, maid-servants, truth, courage, anger, patience, cunning, ears and self-interest.

Fourth: Relations, mother, conveyances, lands, education, happiness, pleasures, wells, tanks, gardens, rivers, doors, books, houses, beds, cows, work, medicines, magic, litigation, witness and holy passages.

Fifth: Children, strength, intelligence, and natural shrewdness.

Sixth: Enemies, pollution, fear, cousins, sins, arms, disease, misery, debt and mental anxiety.

Seventh: Passions, wife, cupidity, sexual pleasures, mercantile speculations, ambassadors, marriage decoration, exchange of commodities, gambling and venereal thoughts.

Eighth: Life, death, destruction, means of livelihood, final emancipation, sin and disease.

Ninth: Merit, teachers, elders, father, kindness, respect for holy beings, worship, divine knowledge, peace and happiness.

Tenth: Respect, reputation, command, work, prosperity, merit, political success, business strength of mind, nervous energy, good deeds.

Eleventh: Longevity, acquisition of wealth, success in life, friends, elder sisters, gain and pleasure.

Twelfth: Waste, sin, hell, heaven and evil deeds.

Here the idea is that if a man wants to know how and when he will be married, the astrologer must fix correctly the birth sign of such a man and all the planets at the time and then he must examine the 7th house from the Lagna or birth sign. If a good planet occupies the 7th or aspects it, if its lord is powerful and joins good house or planets, and is not otherwise debilitated, then the person will have a good and pretty wife and she will be from a respectable family. If he wants to know about his father he must refer to the 9th house from birth. They are called the Dwadasha Bhavas or houses signifying all the events of human life.

❖❖❖

CHAPTER - 7

EARLY DEATH OR BALARISHTA

The readers have already learnt how to fix the lagna and the other planets at the time of birth and I shall take now to an important chapter where you can learn how to ascertain the longevity of a person. There are six divisions in the term of man's life which have been given some prominence by the astrological writers and they are not unimportant. Balarishta is the combination of planets where the child dies before it is 8 years, Madhyarishta details combinations of planets which inflict death after 8 years and before the child passes its 20th year.

Then come the combinations of planets called Yogarishta wherein they kill the youths after 20 and before they pass their 32nd year. Then come the combinations for Alpayu (short life) which take the man beyond the 32nd year, and kill him before he is 50 years. Then come the Madhyayu combinations wherein the person dies between 50 and 76 years. This is called middle life.

Those who manage to live beyond 75 years and up to 120 years are said to enjoy the poornayu combinations or full or long life. The abbreviations are:

Ravi	Sun R.	☉	Shukra	Venus S.	♀
Chandra	Moon C.	☽	Shani (Manda)	Saturn M.	
Kuja	Mars K.	♂	Rahu (Thama)	Dragon's Head T.	☊
Budha	Mercury B.	☿	Ketu	Dragon's Tail Kt.	☋
Guru	Jupiter G.	ψ			

The Abbreviations for the zodiacal signs are				
Aries	♈	Mesha	A.	For Ghatikas Ghts.
Taurus	♉	Vrishabha	Ts.	For Vighatikas VGhts.
Gemini	♊	Mithuna	Gi.	Trimshamsha Tm.
Cancer	♋	Kataka	Cr.	Navamsha N.
Leo	♌	Simha	Lo	Lagna L.
Virgo	♍	Kanya	V.	For Hora H.
Libra	♎	Tula	L.	For Drekkana Dr.
Scorpio	♏	Vrischika	So	For Shashtiamsha Sh.
Sagittarius	♐	Dhanus	Ss.	For periods (Dasha) Ps.
Capricorn	♑	Makara	Cs.	For Sub-periods Sp. (Vidasha)
Aquarius	♒	Kumbha	As.	
Pisces	♓	Meena	P.	

BALARISHTA OR EARLY DEATH

1. If Chandra with evil planets occupies 7, 12, 8 or 1 and is not aspected by good planets occupying other than quadrants, the child will not die early.
2. A child born 48 minutes before sunrise or after sunset, when Chandra's Hora is rising and when evil planets occupy the last Navamsha of any of the signs, will die soon.
3. Evil planets in 1 and 7 and Chandra in any house in conjunction with an evil planet without the aspect of benefics, indicate early death of the child.
4. If weak Chandra occupies 12 with evil planets in 1 and 8, without benefics in quadrants, the child will die soon.
5. There will be death if evil planets occupy 12, 2 and 6 and without any conjunction of good planets.
6. Chandra in any of the quadrants, with evil planets in other quadrants, predicts early death. That is Chandra, Shani Kuja and Ravi in 4 quadrants make the child die early.

7. If the birth falls in Cancer or Scorpio with evil planets in 10, 11, 12, 1 and 2, and with good planets in 4, 5, 6, 7, 8 and 9, the child dies early.

8. **(a)** If Chandra is in 6 or 8 aspected by evil planets but not by good planets, the child dies within a month.

   (b) If such Chandra is aspected by benefic and not by malefic, the child dies before 8 years.

   (c) If such Chandra is aspected by good and evil planets together, the child dies before 4 years.

   (d) If such Chandra is not aspected by any planet, good or evil, the child dies within a month.

9. If good planets are in 3 and 8 aspected by powerful evil planets, the child dies within a month.

10. If the lord of the birth is conquered in the planetary fight (Grahayudha) by an evil planet and occupies 7, the child dies before a month.

11. If a weak Chandra occupies birth sign and evil planets are in 8, 4, 7 and 10, the child dies soon.

12. If Chandra is in 4, 7 or 8 and has two or more evil planets on both sides, the child will have an early grave.

13. Chandra in the birth, evil planets in 2, 12, 7 and 8 without good aspects, will send the child and its mother to an early grave.

14. If Chandra occupies the last navamsha of any sign, and aspected by good planets, and with evil planets in 8 and 9 the child dies soon. There will be danger to the father also.

15. Chandra in birth and evil planets in 7 will kill the child early.

16. If Chandra with Shani, Rahu and Kuja occupy 8th, the child and the mother will die soon.

17. If Ravi with Shani or Budha and with Rahu occupies birth, and Kuja in 8, the child and mother will die by weapons or be killed.

18. Ravi or Chandra in birth, without good aspect and evil planets in 5, 8 and 9, will kill the child and mother.

19. Shani in 12, Ravi in 9, Chandra in birth and Kuja in 8, not aspected by benefics, will kill the child, but if Guru is in 5 and aspects all these powerfully there is no fear for the child.

20. If weak Chandra with malefics, not aspected by good ones occupies 5, 7, 9, 12, 1 or 8, the child dies.

21. If Kuja without good aspect occupies 1, while Shani is in 6 or 8, or if Kuja and Shani together occupy 7 without good aspect, the child dies straightway.

22. Children born while Cancer is passing and Leo rising or Scorpio passing and Sagittarius rising or Pisces passing and Aries rising will not live long.

Here the last half ghatika of passing, and the first half of the rising signs are considered to be unfavourable, and they inflict certain death.

23. If Ravi and Chandra occupy 3, owned and aspected by evil planets, the child dies before 3 years.

24. If Ravi and Kuja occupy 7 from Chandra and the 3 Drekkanas of the birth are occupied by malefics, death comes in 10 days.

25. If a weak Chandra is in birth and the other planets occupy 3, 6 and 12, the child dies.

26. If the lord of birth is weak, with evil planets in birth, children born during eclipses under such combination will die in 2 or 3 months.

27. If Rahu with evil planets, without beneficial aspects, occupies any one of the quadrants, the child dies early.

28. If weak Chandra is with Rahu in birth, aspected by evil planets, the child dies soon. This has two exceptions: (a) When Rahu is in Aries. (b) When Rahu is in Taurus. In these cases there will be sickness, but no danger to life.

29. If Guru is not in 8, the lord of birth is with a malefic aspected by Shani, and an evil planet occupies third sign, the child dies.

30. If Ravi is in 7, Shani in 1, Kuja in 8 and Chandra is not aspected by good planets, the infant dies.

31. If Guru is in Scorpio or Ketu is aspected by Ravi, Chandra, Kuja and Shani, and these are not aspected by Shukra, then the infant is born dead.

32. If Chandra is in the 20th part of Aries (divide the sign into 30 equal parts), 21st of Leo, 8th of Taurus, 22nd of Cancer, 4th of Libra, 20th of Capricorn, 18th of Scorpio, 10th of Pisces, 22nd of Gemini, then the infant dies at the ages respectively denoted by the figures.

33. If Ravi, Shani and Kuja occupy birth, Shukra in 7 and Chandra is weak and not aspected by Guru, the child dies before 7 years.

34. If the lord of birth is in the birth itself with all evil planets unaspected by benefics, the child dies before 4 months.

35. If retrograde Shani occupies Aries or Scorpio and if Kuja is in 6 or 8 or any of the kendras without beneficial aspect, the child dies before 2 years.

36. If a person is born in the Lagna of his father, when the lord of Lagna is between two evil planets without the conjunction of benefics, he will meet an early death.

37. If Rahu is in 7 and is aspected by Shani, Ravi and other evil planets, the child will live up to 12 years.

38. If Aquarius, Scorpio or Leo becomes the birth sign with Rahu in it, aspected by malefics, but not by powerful Guru, the child dies before 17 years.

39. If Ravi, Chandra and Kuja occupy 5 without being in conjunction with or aspected by good planets, the child dies before 9 years.

40. If the lord of the birth occupies 3, 6 or 12 and evil planets occupy 8 and 6 without being aspected by good planets, the boy will not survive his 16th year.

41. If the lord of birth is in 8 and the lord of 8 is in 1, and the lord of 2 occupies 6 or 12, the boy dies in his 18th year.

42. If Ravi, Chandra and Kuja occupy the fifth, without good conjunction, the child dies in his 9th year.

43. If the lord of the house occupied by the Moon is the Sun and the Sun occupies with Saturn, the eighth house from Lagna having good aspects, the child dies in the 12th year.

44. If the lord of Lagna and eighth mutually exchange their houses without conjunction or if they both occupy 6th or 12th house without Jupiter, the child dies at 18.

45. If evil planets occupy quadrants without the aspect of Chandra or other benefics and if Chandra occupies 1st, 6th or 12th house, the child lives up to 20 years.

46. If Chandra joins Shani and Ravi occupies 8th, the child dies before his 9th year.

I have given at considerable length the planetary positions of early death, for without a proper foundation, no superstructure will be permanent or lasting. This is very important. Combinations for early death are not exhausted, nor it is possible to do so in an elementary work like this. The Principal points here seem to be that the birth sign should not be between two evil planets as also the 7th, that Chandra should always have some good aspect, that evil planets should not occupy quadrants without good aspect, that the lord of the birth sign should be well situated and aspected, that good planets should occupy quadrants or trines and that the 8th house and Manda should also be powerful. If these conditions are present then the life of the child will be long.

ANTIDOTES FOR EARLY DEATH

I Shall here state a few combinations which avert the above evil influences for early death and enable the child to tide over early death and live to longer periods.

1. Guru powerfully situated in birth sign will avert all evil. The word 'powerfully' is often used in this work in

connection with planets. It means that the planet should be strong in Shadvargas and must have the other sources of strength named in the astrological works, such as Sthanabala, Kalabala, Chestabala, Exaltation, Moolathrikona and so forth.

2. If the lord of the birth has no evil aspects, it has the aspect of good planets situated in quadrants, there is no danger.
3. Even when Chandra is placed in 8 if he occupies any of the Drekkanas of Guru, Shukra or Budha, there is no danger.
4. Full Chandra in good house, placed between two benefics and aspected by Shukra, will give long life.
5. If Shukra, Budha or Guru is powerfully placed in any one of the quadrants, even in conjunction with evil planets, the child will have good long life.
6. If Chandra is in 6, but occupies any of the Drekkanas of Guru, Budha or Shukra, there is no danger.
7. When Chandra is between two powerful good planets, there is no fear of danger.
8. Even when Chandra is in 6 or 8, if he is full, he will protect the child born during the nights of Full Moon days or the days of the New Moon days.
9. When full Chandra aspects birth sign with Guru in one of quadrants, there is no danger.
10. When Guru, Shukra, full Chandra and strong Budha occupy auspicious houses, Drekkanas or Navamshas, they protect the child's life against all evil influences.
11. If evil planets are in auspicious subdivisions, aspected by good planets, occupying auspicious Navamshas, the child will live long.
12. If any one of the good planets has suffered defeat, and is aspected by another auspicious planet, the child has long life.

In determining good and evil influences, students have to take into account the planetary states, occupations, exaltations, debilitations, positional, diurnal, nocturnal, lateral and temporal strength and then say which planets have the greatest power. If evil planets are stronger, and are unfavourably situated, they give death or prolonged sickness, but if good planets are stronger and are favourably situated, they give health, wealth and long life.

If good and evil are equally balanced, then partly good and partly bad will result. It is always difficult to fix the age of children before they pass their 12th year.

There are three principal sources of danger which generally threaten the lives of young children: **(1)** The sins of the parents or the evil Karma those parents do now, and they had done before; **(2)** Various evil powers (forces) which are enacting the surface of the earth and the regions of the air called Balagrahs and **(3)** The bad karma of the children themselves committed in their previous birth (Poorva Janma Karma) have to be taken into consideration. These three sources of danger have to be constantly watched by the parents or guardians of the children and remedies which are suggested in Astrology and other Dharma Shastras must be performed after knowing precisely the kind of danger which threatens the life, to avert the evil influences.

Medicines, Japas or discharges of concentrated willpower, charities to deserving people, propitiatory ceremonies and suitable Homas are some of the useful remedies suggested to avert these evil influences. The difficulty is to know the sources and intensity of the evil and meet it beforehand by suitable remedies.

MADHYARISHTA

Those who live beyond 8 years and die before they are 20 years, are said to have Madhyarishta. The reader is strongly recommended to go through this portion carefully. Here, the age is roughly given and the student has to reconcile these combinations with the Dashas and Vidashas of the planets at the time of death and also take into consideration the influences of the Gochara or planetary movements at the time of the termination of life.

YOGARISHTA

1. If Keeta Rashi (Scorpio) is Lagna with Ravi and Guru and the lord of the 8th occupies any of the Kendras the boy dies at 22.
2. If Rahu and Chandra occupy the 7th and 8th with Guru, in the Lagna, he will live up to 22.
3. If Shani occupies birth which is owned by his enemies and benefics, are in 3, 6, 9 and 12, the person dies between 26 and 27.
4. If evil planets occupy 1st, 2nd and 8th houses and the benefics are outside the Kendras, the man dies in his 28th year (houses other than 1, 4, 7 and 10 are meant here).
5. If Chandra is between the lord of the 1st and 8th house and Guru is located in the 12th house, death comes to the person between 27 and 32 years.
6. If the lord of the 8th is a malefic aspected by Guru and another evil planet or if the lord of birth is in the 8th house aspected by them, the person will die in his 28th year.
7. If the lord of the 8th is in one of the Kendras and the lord of the birth is weak, the native dies in the 30th year.
8. If any one of the lords of the 1st and 8th occupies the 8th and the other is powerless, death happens between 30 and 32 years.
9. If Saturn occupies the Navamsha of the 8th house with a powerful planet in the Lagna and the benefics are outside the Kendras, there will be death between 30 and 32 years.
10. If the lords of birth and 8th are in Kendras with some planets in the 8th and benefics outside the Kendras, death comes in the 32nd year.

11. If Ravi and Chandra conjoin and occupy any of the Kendras, with the lord of the 8th in a Kendra, with an evil planet in the 8th house and without any planet in the Lagna, the person lives up to 32 years.

12. If the lord of the 1st and the 8th join together and are in conjunction with malefics and occupy the 8th without benefics, death comes in the 27th year.

13. If Chandra occupies the 9th house from Lagna in the reverse order, with the lord of 8th in a Kendra and in conjunction with or aspected by evil planets, and without the combination of or aspect by good planets, the person dies in his 24th year.

14. If the lord of the 8th occupies birth and the lord of birth is weak, the person dies between 30 and 32.

15. If the Moon and the lord of the birth are in Apoklimas and the latter is aspected by evil planets and otherwise powerless, death overtakes him in a similar time.

ALPAYU OR SHORT LIFE

Persons, who live after 32 and die before they are 50 years, are said to enjoy Alpayu or short life and the combinations show the relative ages to which they attain. In the classifications of longevity the ancient Maharishis in India have made very nice distinctions and even in these main divisions there are other minor subdivisions which appear to be very reasonably thought over and arranged. A man who dies at 32 and one who lives up to 50 certainly have different lengths in their lives and these will be indicated in the following conjunctions:

1. If Guru and Shukra occupy Kendras, with lord of the birth in Apoklimas with malefics and the birth takes place in a sandhyakala the person dies in his 36th year, (sandhyakala means 48 minutes after sunset and 48 minutes before sunrise). This will be the twilight when the Sun is not visible but there will still be some light.

2. If Ravi occupies the lagna, an unfriendly house, between two evil planets and is powerless and has not the aspect of benefics, death comes in the 36th year.

3. If Chandra is in Aries or Scorpio, as the birth sign, aspected by evil planets, with good planets occupying other than quadrants, the man dies in his 33rd year.

4. If the lord of 8 be with evil planets, Chandra occupies quadrants, or trines and evil planets aspects 10, the man dies in his 33rd year.

5. If the lord of the birth is in 6 or 8 with the malefics, unaspected by benefics, the man lives up to 45 years.

6. Chandra in a sign of the lord of the birth, powerfully aspected by good planets indicates death in the 47th year after a successful life.

MADHYAYU OR COMBINATIONS FOR MIDDLE AGE

Madhyayu means middle life. Persons, who manage to live beyond 50 years and die before they are 75, are said to enjoy middle life and those who live above 75 and die before they are 120 years are said to enjoy full life. Persons who live above 120 years and to any extent, are said to enjoy unlimited life or Aparimitayurdaya.

1. Shani in birth, Chandra in 8 or 12 and other planets in 11 denote death in the 52nd year.

2. Guru in Sagittarius, it being the birth sign, Kuja and Rahu in 8, kill the man in the 57th year.

3. Chandra with evil planets, and the lord of the 8th in the 7th, kill the man in the 58th year.

4. Aquarius as birth, Guru in 8 and evil planets in the quadrants, make a man charitable, holy, learned, and kill him when he is 60 years.

5. Shani in birth, Chandra in 4, Kuja in 7 and Ravi in 10 with Guru, Shukra and Budha occupying unfavourable houses, give one 60 years of life.

6. Shukra in 10, aspected by Budha, Guru and Chandra, make the man live up to 60 years.
7. Shukra in birth, Budha and Shani in quadrants and other planets exalted, occupy 3 and 11, the person will have a bright life up to 60 years.
8. Ravi with lord of the birth in 10, Shani in the birth sign and Guru in 4, give the person 68 years of life.
9. Birth sign Cancer with Chandra in it, Shani in 8 and Ravi in 7, will give 65 years of life.
10. Shani debilitated occupying quadrants or trines and Budha with Ravi or without him, occupies quadrants, give the person 70 years of life and make him good, charitable and learned.
11. Good planets occupying quadrants, 8th house without any aspect from them and the lord of the birth with the aspect of the evil planets, give a man 70 years of life.
12. With Kuja in 5, Shani debilitated and Ravi in 7, the persons will have 70 years of life span.

POORNAYU OR LONG LIFE

1. All good planets in the first six houses from birth and all bad planets in the next six houses make a man rich, educated, good natured and he lives up to 80 years of age.
2. Benefics in quadrants, 8th unoccupied by evil planets, and Chandra in 6 give the man 86 years of life.
3. Guru in a quadrant from the lord of the birth, without evil planets in quadrants or trines give 100 years of life.
4. If Leo is birth sign, and four planets occupy the trines, the man lives for 100 years.
5. If Taurus or Cancer is birth sign with Guru in it and three planets are exalted, the person lives up to 106 years.
6. Guru exalted in Cancer with birth there and the exaltation of two more planets will be enough to give him long life.

7. Shukra in 4, Guru in birth and Chandra and Shani in 10 give the person long life, good name, high education and moderate wealth.

8. If the birth sign falls in the 2nd half of Capricorn with Kuja in the first half, Chandra in birth sign and Guru occupies one of the quadrants, the person lives for more than hundred years.

9. If the birth time falls in the last Navamsha of Pisces and Chandra is in the 5th Thrimshamsha or Taurus and other planets are exalted, the person lives for 120 years.

APARIMITAYURDAYA OR UNLIMITED TERMS OF LIFE

From time immemorial, we have had historical as well as legendary and religious record, wherein the names of persons are mentioned who have lived for more than 120 years, the age fixed by astrological works for ordinary mankind. The Bible, the Koran, the Buddhistic books and the Hindu Puranas give the names of persons who have lived for hundreds and thousands of years, and all of whom, it would be highly injudicious to say, were purely mythological. If the rules of life are carefully studied and analysed and the circumstances of a man's career are favourable and he possesses an abundant quantity of nervous energy, given by the auspicious planetary combinations at the time of birth, and also secured by his straightforward, contended and jolly temperament, I do not see that such long terms of life are either impracticable or impossible to achieve. In the Encyclopedia Brittanica, some names of persons are found, who have lived quite recently for more than 150 years. It is possible and it would be possible to prolong life beyond the so-called natural limits, if the necessary knowledge of life is carefully understood and the physical and mental conditions are strictly adhered to and practised in conformity with the moral and natural laws.

Unlimited terms of life may look strange to the modern scientists and sceptics, but many of the most eminent men among the former, are now beginning to see the importance of leading simple lives, possessing hopeful temperaments, practising regulated habits and living under very favourable natural psychological conditions. The introspection of the West is an outgrowth of tentative methods, and does not even approach the outer-line of the Yoga of the Hindus — the concentration of mind and its development will give vigour and energy to body and make it least vulnerable to the attacks of human ills. The various other processes recommended in the Yoga for the emancipation of the mind from its numerous gross and physical environments and worries, and the study of Vedas and Vedanta, wherein very sublime subjects are brought in contact with the mind and enable it to grasp the higher intelligence, are not matters at which any deep thinker can afford to take a 'ridiculous laugh'. There are many matters in heaven and earth which we do not know and, at which, as honest men, we should not laugh.

A little practice in them, after proper initiation by a Sadguru (authorised good preceptor) will convince any sensible person of the grand system of knowledge acquired by the Hindu Maharishis in the earliest stages of human existence and used so successfully by them in the investigation of all the recorded sciences in the fields of Aryan literature. This is a matter which cannot be shelved into the Fabulous Regions, as if described by the heated brains or ill-informed persons. A little practice and personal experience will show that life can be prolonged to any extent and taken out of the body at the sweet will of the holder.

1. If birth sign is Cancer with Chandra and Guru there, Shukra and Budha in quadrants and Kuja, Ravi and Shani occupy 3, 6 and 11 respectively, the person lives for a long time.

2. Birth sign Leo with Guru, Shukra in Cancer, Budha in Virgo, evil planets in 3, 6 and 11, the person lives for thousand years.

3. If birth sign is Aries, Ravi in Cancer, Shani in Capricorn, Kuja in Libra, powerful Chandra in Pisces, the person lives for 2000 years.
4. No evil planets in trines, no good planets in quadrants and no evil planets in 8, will make a man live for a long time.
5. Birth sign in Taurus with Shukra and Guru in quadrants and the rest in 3, 6, 10 and 11, will make a man live very long.
6. Birth sign in Cancer, Shani in Libra, Chandra in Taurus, Guru in Capricorn, will give a man very long life.
7. Guru, Shani, Kuja and Shukra must be in quadrants to each other; if so, they give very long life.
8. If birth sign is Leo and Guru, Chandra, Shukra and Budha occupy quadrants, with Ravi, Shani and Kuja in 3, 6 and 11, the person lives for thousand years.

COMBINATIONS FOR YOGA

I shall give here a few combinations for becoming Yogis who live as long as they please, and leave the physical body at their pleasure and will, through the bursting of the upperskull.

1. The seven planets must commence from Cancer and occupy consecutively the following signs, viz., Cancer, Leo, Virgo, Libra, Scorpio and Sagittarius. There should be no break in the middle. Then the person will become a great Yogi and will live a long life.
2. If all the planets are between Chandra and Guru, then the person becomes a Yogi and will live long.
3. If all the planets are between Shani and Kuja the man becomes a Yogi.
4. When Capricorn is the birth sign and all the planets are between Ravi and Kuja, he becomes a great Mahatma.
5. If the birth time is in the last Navamsha of Aries with Guru, or Shukra in Aries, Chandra in 2 and Kuja in

Simhasanamsha or in the 5th Navamsha or Sagittarius, the man becomes a great Mahatma.

6. If Cancer is birth sign with Guru in it, Shani in Libra, Chandra in Taurus, Shukra in Gemini and Ravi and Budha in immovable signs, the person becomes a great Sage.

7. When Chandra occupies Davalokamsha, Kuja in Parvathamsha and Ravi in Simhasanamsha he becomes a Sage.

8. If Aries is birth, Ravi in 10, Guru in Cancer and the rest of the evil planets occupy 3, 6, and 11, the person will have great spiritual excellence. Atma in Sanskrit means the soul. Maha means great and therefore, a Mahatma is one whose soul has been purified and expanded by Yoga and Shastra practices. A Sage is one who has attained to a certain psychic development by his Yoga and Jnana.

❖❖❖

CHAPTER - 8

MISFORTUNES

This Chapter as well as the next one become very important in knowing how time stands with any particular individual, and the precautions given can be taken by those who are interested in their welfare to minimise the evil results indicated by the planetary conjunction, or avert them altogether. In fact, if a careful analysis of human history is made, it will be seen that human intellectuals have always kept up a continuous struggle with the natural forces, for a mastery over them. Their inventions and discoveries bear unmistakable evidence to this struggle and it would be absurd, therefore, to say that the study of any branch of human knowledge will be useless which is able to read the future of man and which gives him a timely warning to meet the threatened dangers and difficulties as best as he could.

This is a very difficult part of the subject and requires a vast amount of knowledge to understand it thoroughly, but nothing is beyond the reach of human intellect and though readers may not grasp many of these difficult ideas in the commencement of their studies, they are sure to understand them later on, provided they have the necessary intelligence and devotion to their subjects. Under the different significations of the signs, I shall give some examples of good and evil influences. To know the evil first and then to take suitable remedies in time, will be a more valuable branch of human knowledge than to waste our energies in inventing enjoyments for weal stomachs and heads and then take the evil consequences with helpless impotency under the false impression of philosophy and resignation. I shall here state some of the most important misfortunes which attack men and bend them thoroughly under their combined weight. Although nobody likes to suffer misfortunes, all mankind are subjected to them in some shape or another. These misfortunes are the results of the violations of the natural laws and principles of right and wrong in the previous states of existence and this is called their Past Karma.

The result of violation of natural laws can be remedied by a proper study of those laws and of the higher forms of energy, which control or modify them. The intensity of the misfortune depends upon the evil nature of the planet and the site it occupies, and when remedies are adopted, they must be suitable to meet the threatened danger. It is simple cowardice to shirk off to acknowledge the future misfortunes. It is mainly to know them and meet them by such remedies, as human genius has discovered for such purposes.

1. Rahu with Lord of 2, in 6, or the lord of the sign where Rahu is placed joins with the lord of 2, the man suffers from constant toothache.
2. If the lord of 2 is with the lord of 6, or lord of the house where the lord of 2 is placed, joins with the lord of the Navamsha where he is placed, then during their periods or sub-periods, the man will have his teeth knocked off.
3. If the lord of 2 is with Shani or with any other evil planet, the person suffers from constant complicated diseases.
4. If Ravi in birth sign occupies a debilitated Navamsha or is in conjunction with malefics, his eyes will be pulled out by incurring the displeasure of the rulers or he will be thrashed.
5. If Shani, Kuja and lord of 2 occupy birth sign or the lords of 2 and 6 occupy birth sign, or Kuja and Gulika occupy 12th house, there will be constant pain in the ears or his ears will be cut off.
6. If Shukra is in 6 and Kuja is in birth sign, the person will have his ears cut off.
7. If Chandra is aspected by Shani and the birth sign is aspected by Ravi and Shukra, unaspected by a benefic, the person will have his ears cut off.
8. If Rahu, Shani and Ravi occupy 7, the man will be bitten by a cobra.

9. If Budha occupies one of the houses of Guru and Kuja occupies one of the houses of Shani, the person will be killed in a jungle by a tiger.
10. If Chandra and Shani occupy one of the houses of Shukra, the person will be killed by a sword.
11. If Kuja is in 9 and Shani and Rahu are in conjunction, the person will be killed by arrows or similar sharp weapons.
12. If Guru is in birth with the lord of the 3rd, there is constant fear from quadrupeds.
13. If the birth sign is a watery one, there is fear from aquatic animals.
14. If debilitated planets occupy 3 and defeated planets occupy 6, without beneficial aspects, there is danger from poison.
15. If 4 is occupied by debilitated and defeated planets and 6 becomes a watery sign, the man will be drowned in tanks, rivers or other watery places
16. If the lord of the birth is powerless and occupies 4 with debilitated Ravi or other evil planets, and the lord of the 4 is weak and is in conjunction with watery planets, the man will have a watery grave.
17. If the lord of 1 and 4 combine and occupy 4 and have the aspect of the lord of 10, the man will have a watery grave.
18. If the lord of the house occupied by the lord of 4 is aspected by or is in conjunction with the lord of 4, he dies by drowning.
19. If Ravi and Kuja are in 4, aspected by or in conjunction with the lord of 4 and 10 the person will be stoned to death or will die by falling on a stone or a stone falling on him.
20. If the lord of 4 is in conjunction with Shani and Rahu, aspected by Kuja without the sign of good planets, the person will die from a similar misfortune.
21. If Virgo is the birth sign with Ravi in it, and Shani in 7, the person will become a widower. Here, though he marries often, he will send all his wives to the grave before he proceeds there himself.

22. If Virgo is the birth, with Ravi in it and Kuja in 5, the man will see all his children dead.

23. If Shani, Kuja and Ravi are in 4 and 8 from Shukra, the wife of the person will be burnt to death before him.

24. If Shukra is between two powerful malefics, the wife of the person will die before him by a fall from an elevated place.

25. If Shukra is not with good planets, or has not their aspects, the man's wife will die from wound inflected by bondages or ropes.

26. If 12 and 6 are occupied–one by Ravi and the other by Chandra, the person, as well as his wife, will have, each, one eye only.

27. If 9 or 5 is occupied by Ravi and Shukra, the person will have a limbless wife, that is, his wife will have some defect in one of her organs.

28. If Shani is in birth sign, with Shukra in the last Navamsha of Cancer, Scorpio, Pisces and occupies 7, while benefics are not in 5, the person's wife will be barren. Here, if he marries a second wife, he will be getting children.

29. When Chandra is in 5 and all malefics are in 7, 12 and 1, the person will have neither wife nor children.

30. If Chandra is in 10, Shukra in 7 and evil planets in 4, the person will lose all his children during his life.

31. If Shukra and Kuja are in 7, aspected by evil planets, the person will be night-blind.

32. If Chandra occupies any one of the Navamshas of Kuja and is in conjunction with evil planets, the person will have some incurable disease in the private organ.

33. If Shukra and Shani are in 12 and 2 respectively, Chandra in birth sign and Ravi in 7, the person will be affected by white leprosy.

34. If Chandra is in 10, Kuja in 7 and Shani in 2 from Ravi, the man will have defective organs.

35. If Chandra is between Kuja and Shani, and Ravi is in Capricorn, the man will be subjected to any one of the following diseases – hard breathing, dyspepsia, consumption, enlargement of glands in the left side of the stomach or enlarged spleen.

36. If Ravi is in Cancer or Chandra is in Leo or if Ravi and Chandra exchange their mutual Navamshas, the person will have consumption.

37. If Chandra occupies the 5th Navamsha of Sagittarius or occupying any one of the signs Pisces, Cancer, Capricorn or Aries, and is aspected by or is in conjunction with Shani or Kuja, the person suffers from leprosy. If Chandra is aspected by good planets, the person suffers from cutaneous eruptions.

38. If Scorpio, Cancer, Taurus and Capricorn become 5th or 9th houses from the birth sign and are aspected by or are in conjunction with evil planets, the man will be affected by leprosy.

39. If Ravi, Chandra, Kuja and Shani in any order occupy 8, 6, 2 and 12, the person will lose his sight by that disease which is attributed to the most powerful among the said planets. Ravi represents heat and fire. Chandra represents cold and watery diseases, Kuja represents life and dangers from weapons and animals, Shani represents windy and cutaneous complaints.

40. If Ravi, Chandra, Kuja and Shani occupy in any order, 9, 11, 3 and 5 without beneficial aspects, the man will become blind by that disease which is attributed to the most powerful among them.

41. If evil planets occupy 7 without the aspect of good ones, the man suffers from toothache.

42. If Chandra with Rahu occupies birth sign and Shani and Kuja occupy trines, the person will be possessed of evil spirits.

43. If Ravi with Rahu occupies 1, and Shani and Kuja are in trines, the man becomes perfectly blind.

44. If Shani is in 7 and Guru is in 1, the person will constantly suffer from flatulence.

45. If Kuja is in 7 and Guru is in 1, the person will suffer from brain disease or mental derangement.

46. If Shani is in 1 and Kuja occupies 5, 9 or 7, the man will suffer a similar derangement.

47. If Chandra with Shani occupies 12, the person will be subjected to a similar complaint.

48. If the lord of the Navamsha occupied by Chandra himself, and Ravi and Guru occupy the Navamshas of the planets in whose house they are debilitated or occupy unfriendly Navamshas, the person will become a slave. Here, there are 3 kinds: **(1)** If one of the planets occupies such a position, the man will sell himself for food **(2)** if two planets occupy such positions, he will be sold as a slave by others and **(3)** if three or more planets occupy such positions, he will be born for slave parents.

49. If Taurus, Aries or Scorpio, is birth sign with malefic aspects, the person will have very ugly teeth.

50. If Sagittarius, Taurus, Aquarius, Leo or Capricorn, becomes the birth sign aspected by evil planets, the man becomes baldheaded with uncouth appearance.

51. If Ravi is in 5 or 9 aspected by evil planets, he will be born blind or will have defective sight.

52. If Shani occupies 5 or 9 possessing evil aspects, the person will suffer from a host of complicated diseases.

53. If Kuja occupies 5 or 9 aspected by evil planets, the person will suffer from a loss of limbs or will have defective organs.

54. If birth sign is Aries, Taurus or Sagittarius and evil planets, occupy, in any order, 5, 2, 9 and 12, the person will be imprisoned and fastened by stout ropes or chains.

55. If birth sign is Gemini, Virgo, Libra or Aquarius and evil planets occupy 2, 5, 9 and 12 in order, the man will be heavily chained and imprisoned.

56. If birth sign falls in Cancer, Capricorn or Pisces and malefics occupy 5, 2, 6 and in any order, the person will be imprisoned and chained in an inaccessible town or place.
57. If Scorpio is birth sign with evil planets in 2, 5, 9 and 12, the man will be confined in an unwholesome underground dungeon.
58. If Chandra is with Shani, the man becomes a quarrelsome fellow.
59. If Chandra is with Shani and aspected by Kuja, he becomes an idiot.
60. If Chandra has the ring round him at the time of birth, joined by Shani and aspected by Kuja, he will suffer from consumption.
61. If Ravi, Kuja and Shani are in 10 without beneficial aspects, the person becomes a coolie. When one of the above planets is in 10, without the aspect of good planets, the person becomes a chief among coolies, or cooly maistry.
62. When two planets occupy 10 without good aspect the man will be an ordinary coolie.
63. When there are 3 planets without good aspect in 10, he becomes a coolie of the lowest class.
64. If Kuja is in 8 with Shani, or aspected by him, the person will have his head cut off in battle.
65. If Capricorn or Aquarius is birth sign with Rahu in it, or is in Leo, the person will lose his head in battle.
66. If the lord of the 6th joins birth with a malefic or occupies 8th with evil aspects, there will be sores or wounds.
67. If there is a malefic in 6 and is powerfully aspected by malefics, the person will suffer from sores.
68. If Kuja, Budha and birth lord combine in the 4th, or 12th there will be disease in the anus, jaundice or leprosy.
69. If Chandra, Budha and birth lord join with the Sun and Rahu, there will be venereal disease.
70. If Chandra, Budha and birth lord occupy the Simha navamsha, there will be venereal disease.

71. If Chandra, Budha and birth lord combine with Kuja, there will be leprosy, and if they join with Shani, there will be black leprosy.

72. If Chandra, Budha and birth lord join Ravi, the person will suffer from bloody disease.

73. If the lords of 1st and 6th combine:

(a) with Ravi, there will be danger from fever;

(b) with Chandra, there will be danger from water;

(c) with Kuja, there will be danger from weapons or smallpox or fire;

(d) with Budha, there will be bilious complaints;

(e) with Shukra, there will be danger to wife;

(f) with Shani, there will be windy complaints;

(g) with Rahu or Ketu, there will be danger from thieves, headaches and windy complaints.

74. If Budha joins the lord of the 6th and occupies birth, there will be disease in the sexual organ and if Shani joins the 6th lord and is in birth, the sexual organ will be cut or operated upon.

75. If the lord of the 7th joins Shukra and occupies 6th, the wife will be impotent.

76. If the lords of 1st and 6th join Shani and occupy Kendras or Konas, there will be imprisonment. If they join Rahu or Ketu and occupy quadrants or trines, similar results must be foretold.

77. If Shani is in 9 and Guru occupies 3, or if Shani joins 8 and Guru is in 12, his hands will be cut off.

78. If Chandra occupies, 7 or 8 and joins Kuja or Guru, his hands will be cut off.

In these cases, good aspects and exaltations prevent this misfortune. Hands may be cut off or they may become rotten or useless by paralysis and other nervous complaints.

79. If 10th is occupied by Rahu, Shani and Bhuda, his hands will be cut off.

80. If the lord of the 6th joins Shukra while Shani or Ravi joins with Rahu and occupies cruel subdivisions, the person will have his head cut off.

81. If Chandra occupies 6, 8 or 12 having the aspect of the lord of birth and joins Shani, Rahu and Mandi the person dies by accident.

82. If the lord of the 8th is found in Pasha or Sarpa Drekkanas, the person will die from imprisonment or hanging.

83. If the lord of the Drekkana occupied by the lord of the 8th joins Shani, Rahu or Mandi, there will be death by hanging.

84. If the lord of 6th or 8th or Kuja joins with the lord of the 3rd, and combines with Shani and Rahu in cruel divisions, the person will die in a battle.

85. If the lord of the Drekkana occupied by Shani, joins Martian sign or Navamsha and has his aspect, the man dies in battle.

86. If Ravi and Kuja occupy each other's signs or have mutual aspects or occupy each others Navamshas, the person dies in a duel.

87. If there are many malefics in the 8th and these malefics occupy Martian and cruel subdivisions, the person will die with many others.

88. If all benefics are in debilitation or combust and occupy unfriendly houses, being defeated in the planetary fight, occupy evil divisions and join with malefics, the person will be put to death by irritated crowds or mobs.

89. If Shani, Rahu and Ravi have the aspect of the lord of the 12th and join cruel divisions, being combust, the person dies with many others.

90. If Ravi occupies 6th and lord of the 6th is with a malefic and Ravi has evil aspects, the person suffers from bilious complaints.

91. If Chandra occupies 6th with evil aspects and in cruel divisions, the person will have windy complaints.

92. If Kuja is in 6 with evil aspects and occupies evil divisions, the person will suffer from bloody and bilious ailments.

93. If Budha is in 6 with malefic aspects and bad amshas, (divisions) the man ails from phlegmatic complaints.

94. If Chandra and Kuja are in 6, the man will have cholera or white jaundice. If Chandra joins Ravi and occupies 6th, the persons will have plague, cholic or some other serious stomach disorder.

95. If Budha and Kuja occupy 6th, aspected by Shukra and Chandra, the person suffers from consumption.

96. If Shani and Kuja are in 6 aspected by Ravi and Rahu, the person will have asthma and consumption.

97. If the powerless lord of the 7th or Kuja occupies birth he suffers from dyspepsia, facial disease, enlarged spleen, or other bilious complaints.

98. If the lord of the Navamsha occupied by the lord of the 6th happens to be Ravi or Kuja, the person suffers similarly.

99. If Chandra is in 6, Shani in 8 and malefic in 12, and lord of birth occupies an evil Navamsha, the person suffers from nasal disease.

100. If the lord of the 9th occupies 6th and the lord of the 6th joins with Kuja and Shani and aspects him, the person will suffer from thieves and fires.

There are many more combinations treating on this important question, but in a small book like this, I cannot exhaust such important subjects.

In all these cases those organs will be afflicted which are indicated by the signs and the planets, and at the times, when the periods and sub-periods of those planets intervene.

❖❖❖

CHAPTER - 9

PLANETS IN THE HOUSES

The significance of the planets in different houses is given here. I have made the language and symbols as concise and simple as possible with a view to make the book handy, and when the planets are marked against the numbers it means that planets in those houses produce the results therein marked.

RAVI (SUN)

Ravi in 1: Bilious, short-sighted, lazy in the transaction of work, intelligent, fond of daring deeds, hot constitution, generally healthy in afterlife, unkind to fellow creatures, successful in political life, careless of reputation, danger from fever in the 3rd year after birth, capricious, if the birth sign is Aries with Ravi there, the person becomes very wealthy and will have a little defective sight. If the birth sign is Leo with Ravi there, the person will be night-blind; if Cancer, the person will have some mole or mark in the eyes, and if Libra, the person will be born blind and poor.

Ravi in 2: Ugly or disfigured face, losses from prosecutions or fires, misappropriation of Government property, angry, stubborn, danger in the 25th year from losses, if aspected by good planets, there will be much wealth and good education, good eyesight, otherwise the sight will be defective.

Ravi in 3: Courageous, famous, intelligent man, cousins, few brothers, wealthy and successful life, danger in the 5th year from quadrupeds.

Ravi in 4: Defective organs, much anxiety, hater of relations, success in a foreign country, short life for mother, heated constitution, very successful in the 22nd year, quarrelsome, unhappy, good reputation.

Ravi in 5: Poor, childless or few children, heart disease, stout, danger to father in the 7th year, indifferent to caste prejudices, corpulence.

Ravi in 6: Intelligent, careless of caste distinctions, warlike, bold, licentious, family composed of children and grandchildren, easy victory over foes, wealthy, eye disease during the 20th year, in afterlife, great gains from former enemies.

Ravi in 7: Man of loose morals, hated by the fair sex, late marriage, submissive to wife, fond of travelling, acquisition of wealth through female agency, fond of eating in others' houses, wife's character rather questionable, if good planets aspect, she will be virtuous, fair and will have erect and strong breast, bilious in temperament, two wives, eating things prohibited by his caste.

Ravi in 8: Few children, long life, complaint in eyes, sores in the head in the 10th year, weak constitution, uncharitable.

Ravi in 9: Fond of sublime subjects, charitable, godly, little wealth, few children, little patrimony, self-acquired property, many lands, glandular disease.

Ravi in 10: Famous, clever in the art of acquiring wealth, superior knack, healthy, educated, highly courageous, fond of music, fine taste, good children, founder of villages or colonies, commanding much personal influence, successful military or political career.

Ravi in 11: Much wealth, many vehicles, steady and persevering in any undertaking, good reputation, many political enemies, man of principles, healthy.

Ravi in 12: Poor, thief, adulterous among widows, tall persons, unscrupulous conduct, careless of reputation.

CHANDRA (MOON)

Chandra in 1: Handsome, but sickly stout body, flatulence, disease in private organs and ears, educated, many brothers, fits, mental derangement, stubborn, danger from drowning. In Cancer, Chandra makes a man wealthy, in Aries, Chandra gives many children, in Taurus, Chandra gives excellent position and great wealth.

Chandra in 2: Handsome, countenance, charming eyes, highly intelligent, wealthy, breaks in education, great respect in government, good family, sweet speech.

Chandra in 3: Dyspeptic complaint, piles, not suckled by mother, fine sisters, thin, body, impious, many brothers, educated, courageous, cruel.

Chandra in 4: Fine taste, high education, polite manners, good houses, horses, and furniture, many relations, much wealth, happy, licentious, protector of many persons, good mother.

Chandra in 5: Many horses and cattle, handsome wife, shrewd, showy, imperfect education, many daughters.

Chandra in 6: Lazy, submissive to females, tender body, weak sexual connection, fond of widows, poor, drunkard, pilfering habits, suckled by strangers, imperious, intelligent, weak stomach, many foes.

Chandra in 7: Fond of women, blood thirsty, handsome wife, good family, pain in the loins. When aspected by evil planets, two wives, narrow minded, jealous, full of sexual energy.

Chandra in 8: Unsteady, unhealthy, few children, mother short lived, maternal disagreement, bilious, lean body, and sight defective.

Chandra in 9: Lover of stories, intelligent, builder of tanks, temples and charitable places, good children, godly, many lands, gold, popular, friends, relations, wealthy.

Chandra in 10: Charitable, bold, shrewd, enjoying the fruits of his labour, fond of widows, adulterous, business tact, long life, successful, respect for elders and priests, wealthy.

Chandra in 11: Well informed, philanthropic, literary taste, polite, wealthy, good cultivation, charitable, man of principles.

Chandra in 12: Mean habits, constantly hearing of evil news, many relations, defective organs, narrow minded, cruel.

KUJA (MARS)

Kuja in 1: Burn or scar in the body, over-heated constitution, thievish habits, corpulence good complexion, respected, danger to father.

Kuja in 2: Short temper, extravagant and immoral, breaks in education, large patrimony in lands and jewels.

Kuja in 3: Few brothers, intelligent, very bold, adulterous as also the wife if aspected by evil planets, fond of dancing girls, adventurous, unpopular, many cousins.

Kuja in 4: Danger to parents, sickly mother, family quarrels, good conveyances, dependent on others, brutal, tyrannical in the treatment of women.

Kuja in 5: Childless, incurring government displeasure, unpopular.

Kuja in 6: Wealthy, good lands, conquest over enemies, good political life, intelligent, secret enemies.

Kuja in 7: Sickly wife, passing blood or suffering from piles, disease in hands, many brothers and maternal uncles, intelligent.

Kuja in 8: Few issues, bad sight, short life, danger to father, good father and maternal uncles, fond of dancing women, widower in afterlife.

Kuja in 9: Loss from cultivation, sickly father, cruel disposition, dependent life, merchandise in boats and ships and gains thereby.

Kuja in 10: Clever in getting wealth, sound health, famous, founder of towns or colonies, self-acquired properly, good cultivation and profit.

Kuja in 11: Well informed many lands, very shrewd in business, many elder brothers, self-acquired property.

Kuja in 12: Poor rotten body, cheat, unpopular, loss of wife, if with Ketu, incendiary habits.

BUDHA (MERCURY)

Budha in 1: Learned, well informed, fond of magic and astronomy, able to exercise spirits, fond of mathematics and poetry, respected long life.

Budha in 2: Many issues, religionist, sweet speech, wealthy, self-acquired property, fond of storing grain, steady in gaining his object.

Budha in 3: Happy, fortunate in women, many brothers, often cruel.

Budha in 4: Learned, intelligent mother, skilled in the sleights of hand, polite, obliging, careless in keeping carriages and animals, wanting in taste.

Budha in 5: Danger to maternal uncles, sickly parents, political respect, quarrelsome; showy, fond of cloths of all kinds.

Budha in 6: Breaks in education, foeless, respectable, short tempered, cunning, danger to mother, losses in money, disease in toes and fingers.

Budha in 7: Skilled in religious lore, happy mother, many carriages and horses, good health, adulterous, charitable.

Budha in 8: Respectable, long life, obliging, few issues, many lands.

Budha in 9: Obliging, fond of musical instruments, highly licentious, pretending to be holy, many issues.

Budha in 10: Fortunate, enjoyment in life, founder of charities, good name, intelligent performing sacrifices, bad sight, renouncing worldly pleasures in afterlife.

Budha in 11: Many lands, wealth, happiness, mathematical faculty.

Budha in 12: Intelligent, adulterous, capricious, obliging, danger to mother, few children, living in other's houses.

GURU (JUPITER)

Guru in 1: Learned, grammarian or philologist, many children, political success, long happy life, great respect, skilful in various arts, stout and majestic body, golden locks and eyes.

Guru in 2: Handsome person, charming eyes, intelligent, wealthy, eloquent, good wife and family, witty and humorous in conversation, enjoyable in life, great influence among relations.

Guru in 3: Many brothers, misery, polite professions, unscrupulous of the means employed in gaining his object, favourable to cultivation, protecting only very close relations.

Guru in 4: Happy, wealthy, educated, good carriages and horses, helper of relations, fond of building houses, good mother, many cattle.

Guru in 5: Handsome and broad eyes, ministers, divan or commander, few children, very intelligent, skilful in mercantile work, eclipsed by the success of his son.

Guru in 6: Many cousins and good children, foeless, witty, and humorous, licentious, dyspeptic or weak digestion.

Guru in 7: Eclipsing his father in wealth and success, rich marriage, very sensitive, fond of good name, success in cultivation; if aspected by evil planets, wife faithless.

Guru in 8: Mean minded, drunkard, widower, pains in stomach, teacher of servants, pretending to be charitable and misappropriating such funds, long life, dirty habits.

Guru in 9: Benevolent, god-fearing, many issues, performing many religious sacrifices, wealthy, long life to father, educated.

Guru in 10: Learned, clever in the acquisition of wealth, great respect, many lands, good vehicles and horses, many children, governor of villages, many servants and maids, steady and paying cultivation.

Guru in 11: Professor of music, horse and elephants, very wealthy, charitable and god-fearing, dependant, elder brothers.

Guru in 12: Cruel, poor, few issues, connection with women and prostitutes, enlargement of spleen glands, displaying great taste in selection of beds, cots, women and modes of enjoyment of life, Charitable among deserving, members, sanyasi, pious in afterlife.

SHUKRA (VENUS)

Shukra in 1: Mathematician, long life, fond of wife, jewels, clothes, scents, flower and women, skilled in the art of sexual enjoyment.

Shukra in 2: Handsome, large and fair eyes, big family, luxurious food, charming wife, happy, hater of women, fond of fine arts, obliging, agreeable manners, educated, author and poet.

Shukra in 3: Many prospering brothers, obliging, but not spending money, healthy.

Shukra in 4: Good eater, learned, intelligent, kind mother, many cattle and horses, fond of milk, relatives, land and cultivation, successful, popular, famous.

Shukra in 5: Intelligent, statesmanly ability, danger to mother, commander educated, many children chiefly daughters.

Shukra in 6: Foeless, many cousins, very licentious, constant venereal complaints, grand children, well informed, fond of women of all kinds.

Shukra in 7: Skilled in the art of adultery, fond of women, adopting questionable means to gain his ends, thoroughly licentious, wealthy, enjoying sexual pleasure; if with Shani, the wife will also be faithless.

Shukra in 8: Happy, danger to mother, celebrated, short life, wealthy till the end of life, godly in afterlife, unscrupulous in the commencement, pious before death.

Shukra in 9: Religious, respect for elders, commander of infantry, sharp in business, fond of teachers and priests.

Shukra in 10: Breaks in education, god-fearing, few elder brothers, good horses and vehicles, success in the legal line.

Shukra in 11: Learned, wealthy, many lands and much cultivation, good conveyances.

Shukra in 12: Fond of low women, misery, wealthy, sweet promises and sad performances.

SHANI (SATURN)

Shani in 1: Loss of children, evil-natured, unscrupulous; incurring king's displeasure, bad citizen, insignificant life, flatulence, adultery among low women, fond of drinks, if the birth sign is Libra, Sagittarius, Capricorn, Aquarius and Pisces with Shani in it, the person commands respect, wealth, becomes a presidency or town magistrate, educated and of comely appearance though dark.

Shani in 2: Losing wealth, two wives, few lands, diseased face, break in education, adulterous, drunkard, stammering.

Shani in 3: Loss of brothers, polite, obliging, cruel-hearted, many servants, courageous, fond of ladies, good cultivation.

Shani in 4: Two mothers, cholic pains, miserable not open-hearted, fond of oily seeds and dark grains, political disfavour, good patrimony, success in foreign countries, incestuous or prohibited intercourse.

Shani in 5: Issueless, adoption, evil-minded, tale bearer, village life, criminal prosecution; when this sign is common, he is sure to have an adopted son.

Shani in 6: Few cousins, deafness, stubborn, fearless, wealthy, few issues, quarrelsome, fond of women, suffering from complicated diseases.

Shani in 7: Sickly, many wives, fond of prostitutes, travelling, sponge, cheat, cholic pain in ears. In conjunction with Shukra, the wife also becomes unchaste.

Shani in 8: Long sexual organ, corpulent, poor, adultery with low caste women, drunkard, service, work, few children, bad sight, leprosy, expansion of glands, seducing family women. With Shukra travelling and adulterous, with Kuja danger by drowning, with Rahu danger by weapons or poison, with Ravi and Rahu impious, not performing paternal ceremonies, ever thinking of adultery, hard breathing, passing blood, consumption, asthma, few brothers, scandals in wife's family, dishonestly earned money, worthless sons, long life.

Shani in 9: Misery, wearing torn or old garments, constructing tanks, chattarams, temples, danger to paternal aunts, irreligious, unfilial.

Shani in 10: Bathing in the Ganges and other holy rivers, bilious, fond of agriculture, village or town magistrate, misery, forsaking his own country, head or religious institution or Sanyasi.

Shani in 11: Exceedingly wealthy, many lands, great political respect, breaks in education, no elder brothers or paternal uncles, good horses and vehicles.

Shani in 12: Learned, defective organs, skilful in arts, squint eyes, giving money for evil purpose, if with an evil planet, danger to eyes.

RAHU (DRAGON'S HEAD)

Rahu in 1: Childless, abortions, courageous, if he is in Aries, Taurus, Gemini, Cancer, Leo, Virgo and Capricorn results are not so unfavourable.

Rahu in 2: Healthy growth, little wealth, bad sight, loss of children, wives, short temper, close-fisted, fond of drinks.

Rahu in 3: Millionaire, few issues, bold, many brothers, adventurous and warlike, many cousins, ear pains.

Rahu in 4: Breaks in education, fond of foreign languages, many jewels and clothes, two wives, a willing subordinate, two mothers; with Shukra, incestuous intercourse.

Rahu in 5: Loss of children, vomiting disease, cruel-hearted, getting into hot water with superiors, displeasure of government, residence in insignificant villages.

Rahu in 6: Loss in women, wealthy, foeless, many cousins, fond of low caste women, venereal disease, happy.

Rahu in 7: Two wives, 1st wife suffering from passing large quantities of blood, 2nd wife from dyspepsia or enlarged spleen, adultery among widows, diabetes, fond of drinks.

Rahu in 8: Mean-minded, quarrelsome, danger in the 32nd year if in conjunction with evil planets, death in the 56th year if with good planets, immoral.

Rahu in 9: Impious, uncharitable, careless of the future, submissive to women, few children, good subordinate, drunken habits.

Rahu in 10: Connection with widows, wealthy man of fine state, fond of poetry, painting and dramas, traveller, disease from flatulence.

Rahu in 11: Many friends, elder sisters and brothers, adulterous, good civilisation, many children of strong gain.

Rahu in 12: Misery, few children, defective vision, money losses.

KETU (DRAGON'S TAIL)

Ketu in 1: Pains in loins, leprous, palms, emaciated figure, weak constitution, graceless manners, disease from poisonous effects, excessive heat, piles, fond of women, intelligent.

Ketu in 2: Short temper, but sweet tongue, cruel heart, breaks in education, strict in money matters.

Ketu in 3: Very popular, adventurous, many relations, no younger brothers, fond of gems, wealthy.

Ketu in 4: Complaint from poison, quarrelsome, weak, sickly mother, licentious.

Ketu in 5: Tender head, liberal, sinful, eldest issue would be female, loss of children, fond of drinks and women.

Ketu in 6: Rise in the long run, agreeable conversation, admired by women, licentious, venereal disease.

Ketu in 7: Connection with maid-servants, or women serving as sweepers, nurses and attendants, very passionate, sickly wife, committing secret sins, searches after widows.

Ketu in 8: Sanguine, little intelligence, bad eyes, few children, senseless quarrels, ruin to women.

Ketu in 9: Blind or short-sighted, impious, liar, blessed with children, relations and friends.

Ketu in 10: Jolly, enjoying life in all its phases, relations, baths in the Ganges and other holy rivers.

Ketu in 11: Many friends, wealthy, intelligent, courageous, respect among all classes.

Ketu in 12: Fickle-minded, bad sight, residence in a foreign country, low favourites, constant travelling, forsaking native country, obtaining final emancipation or Moksha.

❖❖❖

CHAPTER - 10

RAJAYOGA OR COMBINATION FOR SOVEREIGNTY

I shall briefly point out a few combinations which give royal power. In some of these conjunctions, the power will be attained only by those who are born in royal families, and in others, persons born in the midst of poverty and destitution, rise to kingly power by their own perseverance and energy. Such distinctions are indicated in their suitable places.

Here, combinations for royalty are sketched. There are many persons who are not royal literally, but who wield the royal power. In a Constitutional Government, the king or queen has almost no royal power, as no independent political act could be done by them. The President of Republics or Confederated States are more powerful in some cases. By royalty we have to understand political power and whoever possesses it, will be entitled to such name although these names differ in different countries and at different times and forms of Government.

1. If Ravi, Guru, Shani and Kuja are exalted, and one of the places of their exaltation becomes birth sign, the person becomes a king irrespective of birth and its surroundings.
2. If three planets are exalted, the person becomes an inborn in royal families, otherwise he becomes a great statesman or equal to a king.
3. If Budha, Guru and Shani are exalted with birth, placed in any one of their exalted houses, the person gains sovereignty.
4. If Guru, Shani and Kuja are exalted with the Lagna placed in any one of the houses of their exaltation, he achieves a kingdom.
5. If Ravi, Guru and Kuja are exalted, with the Lagna in any of them, the person becomes a king or his equal in power. In all these cases, if the exalted planets are possessed of evil aspects, the person becomes a bad and tyrannical

ruler or statesman, if aspected by benefics, the person becomes a good and popular prince or ruler.

6. If Ravi and Guru are exalted and Chandra is in Cancer, with birth sign in Aries or Cancer, the man will be a king.
7. If birth is in Aries, Cancer or Libra and Ravi, Chandra and Shani are exalted or if Ravi and Kuja are exalted with Chandra in Cancer and with birth in Aries, Capricorn or Cancer, the person becomes a king.
8. If Guru and Chandra are in Cancer and Kuja is in Capricorn with birth sign in them, or if Guru and Chandra are in Cancer and Shani is in Libra with birth sign in them, the child becomes a monarch.
9. If Chandra is in Cancer, Shani in Libra and Kuja in Capricorn, the person becomes a king, if born in a royal family, otherwise a great man.
10. If birth is in Aries with Ravi in it and Chandra in Cancer or birth in Cancer with Chandra and Guru in it or birth in Libra with Kuja and Chandra in Cancer or birth in Capricorn with Kuja and Chandra in Cancer, the person becomes a king, if he belongs to a royal family or great and influential man if born in other families.
11. If the Vargottama navamsha of any sign of Chandra is aspected by four or more planets, the person becomes a mighty king.
12. If the birth sign is in Aquarius, Aries or Taurus and Shani in Aquarius, Ravi in Aries, Chandra in Taurus, Budha in Gemini and Kuja in Scorpio, the person becomes a king.
13. If Shani and Shukra are in Libra, Chandra in Taurus, Budha and Ravi in Virgo, Guru in Cancer, Kuja in Aries with birth in Libra or Taurus or if Shani and Kuja in Capricorn and Ravi and Chandra are in Sagittarius, the man becomes a powerful king.
14. If Capricorn is birth with Kuja and Chandra in it and Ravi is in Sagittarius, or if Aries is birth with Ravi in it, Chandra and Shani in Libra, Guru in Sagittarius, the person becomes a monarch.

15. If Taurus is birth with Chandra in it or in Leo, Guru in Scorpio, Shani in Aquarius or if Capricorn is birth with Shani in it, Chandra in Pisces, Kuja in Gemini, Budha in Virgo, Guru in Sagittarius; or Pisces is birth with Shukra in it, Guru and Chandra in Sagittarius, Kuja in Capricorn, Budha in Virgo or if Virgo is birth with Budha in it, Guru and Chandra and Kuja in Capricorn and Shukra in Pisces, in all these cases, the person becomes a great king if born in royal families, or a great statesman and wealthy, if born in other families.

16. If Virgo is birth with Budha in it, Shani and Kuja in Capricorn, Chandra and Guru in Sagittarius, the person becomes a great ruler even when born in poor families.

17. If Pisces is birth with Chandra, Shani in Aquarius, Kuja in Capricorn, Ravi in Leo, or if Aries is birth with Kuja, Guru in Cancer, the man becomes a ruler even when he is born in a poor family.

18. If Cancer is birth with Guru, Ravi in Aries, Chandra and Budha in Taurus or if Capricorn is birth with Shani, Kuja in Aries, Chandra in Cancer. Ravi in Leo, Budha in Gemini, Shukra in Libra or if Virgo is birth with Budha in it, Shukra in Gemini and Chandra and Guru in Pisces, Shani and Kuja in Capricorn, or if birth is Aries with Ravi in it, Chandra and Kuja in Capricorn, Guru in Sagittarius, Shani in Aquarius, the person becomes a king if born in royal families, otherwise he will become a great politician and an eminent statesman.

19. If Aries is birth, Ravi in Taurus, Chandra in Libra and other planets in any order in Aquarius, Sagittarius and Aries or if Cancer is birth, Shukra in Libra, Chandra in Pisces and other planets in any order in Virgo, Cancer and Taurus or if powerful Budha occupies birth sign, Shukra or Guru in 9, and other planets in any order in 2, 3, 6, 9, 10, 11, the person becomes a king if born in royal families, or else a great man and he will be benevolent, wealthy and famous.

20. If Taurus is birth with Chandra, Guru in Gemini, Shani in Libra, Ravi, Kuja, Budha and Shukra in Pisces or Chandra in 10, Shani in 11, Guru in birth sign, Budha and Kuja in 2, Shukra and Ravi in 4, the person becomes a great king or statesman as the case may be.

21. Kuja and Shani in birth, Chandra in 4, Guru in 7, Shukra in 9, Ravi in 10, Budha in 11, will make a person of the royal family a king, any other man an exalted statesman.

A few observations will be made here to enable the student to guide him in making predictions as to the exact time when a person may get kingly power, and the time when he may lose it. The planets in the birth sign or those in the 10th will influence the man to get royal power. Suppose there are two or more planets in each of these houses, then find out the strongest planet and predict success during his Dasha or Vidasha. When there are no planets in 1 or 10, the kingdom will be acquired when the sub-period of the most powerful planet arrives. As for the loss of the royal power, the period of the planet occupying an unfriendly house, or who is debilitated must be fixed as that during which the person gets dethroned. If the planets are really powerless to take away the royal power altogether, but if they are partly powerful they give him a temporary banishment or loss of power and then, by means of friendly help, from other rulers, enable him to regain his kingdom.

If Taurus, Cancer, Gemini, Virgo, Sagittarius and Pisces are occupied by good planets, and form Quadrants and the remaining signs owned by evil planets are occupied by their lords, the person will become a great leader of dacoits or robbers and will have wealth and personal influence with many.

We have to make a nice distinction between the leader of a large band of dacoits, and the leader of a small army whose soldiers are also dacoits in a milder sense—who imagines that he has a right to lead armies and acquire kingdoms. From the commencement, the leader of the dacoits feels he is doing something which is not very honourable and the leader of an army feels that he has a fancied right and that his wars are his legitimate work. There is not a wide gulf between the two states, for a powerful leader of daring dacoits, when sufficiently strong, proclaims himself a sovereign and his descendants henceforth have a legitimate claim to succeed to the throne which has been established by the first successful leader.

One great difference, however, between the leader of dacoits and that of an aspiring man to establish a new dynasty of kings, seems to be the intention on the part of the dacoit master to rob the people without reference to their condition and enrich himself and his faithful band of followers, while the man, who aspires for royalty, has got a definite idea of protecting the people and establishing his lawful authority over them. Of course, we have seen in history great tyrants who lived, to plunder the people and violate at every turn, all principles of justice and royal power; but even they pretended to introduce measures for the benefit of their subjects, however mistaken they may be in their views. The dacoit on the other hand makes no pretence whatever to protect the people whom he has robbed. The distinction between dacoits and tyrannical rulers is delicate and requires careful discussion.

CHAPTER - 11

JUDGEMENT OF THE BHAVAS

FIRST HOUSE

1. If the lord of the birth is exalted, well-associated, occupies quadrants, has the aspect of good planets, is in his own or his friendly Navamsha, the man will have health, majestic appearance, great command and general happiness.
2. If the lord of the birth is debilitated, has evil conjunction, or aspect, is weak or occupies unfavourable Navamshas, the person will have bad health, emaciated body, constant sickness and general misery.
3. If evil planets are in birth with Rahu, or if the lord of the birth is in conjunction with malefics, the person will be often cheated and will suffer from thieves and robbers.
4. If the lord of the Navamsha, occupied by the lord of the birth, is in conjunction with Rahu, Kuja, Shani or any one of them, when powerful, the person will have enlarged testicles or hydrocele; if Rahu is with the lord of the Navamsha occupied by the lord of the birth house, there will be a similar complaint.
5. If Kuja and the lord of the birth are together in it with evil planets or have their aspects, the person will have a scar or a cut in the head, will fall from or against a rock or receive some cuts from sharp weapons.
6. If birth is occupied by good planets, aspected by good, but not by evil planets, the person will be stout, if the birth happens to be a watery sign like Cancer or Pisces.
7. Ravi in birth aspected by Kuja gives asthma, consumption, dyspepsia or enlarged spleen. Kuja in birth aspected by Ravi or Shani gives sword cuts; Ketu in birth aspected by malefics gives nightmares, fear of devils, hobgoblins and troubles from thieves.

8. If birth is movable sign, with its lord in a similar sign, the person becomes a great traveller. If birth is movable, its lord in a movable Navamsha and the lord of this Navamsha is in a movable sign aspected by a planet in another movable sign, he becomes a great traveller, and acquires immense wealth in foreign lands.

9. If malefics join or aspect birth, Rahu is in 10, or debilitated planet occupies birth aspected by Ravi, the person becomes unpopular, cruel and unhappy.

10. Good planets in birth, malefics in 2 and quadrants and the lord of the birth is in good Navamsha, the person suffers poverty in the commencement and gains much wealth and good position in afterlife.

11. If Rahu, Shani or Kuja is with the lord of the birth, he may suffer from eye complaints. If Budha joins the lord of the birth and is in 6, he will have eye disease.

12. If Budha is the lord of the birth and is in a quadrant, exaltation or in good conjunction, he becomes charitable eloquent, protector of large families with good sight.

SECOND HOUSE

1. If guru is with the lord of 2 or the latter is aspected or Budha or Shukra occupies good houses, the person becomes a powerful speaker, rich man, protector of families and commands many.

2. If the lord of 2 is debilitated or is joined or aspected by malefics, and the lord of birth is weak, he becomes poor and helpless.

3. If the lord of 2 is exalted, occupies one of the quadrants or trines and the lord of the house where the owner of 2 is placed also occupies quadrants, the person commands money.

4. If the lord of 2 is exalted and aspected by or is in conjunction with Guru, he protects thousands of people.

5. If the lord of 2 is in a quadrant aspected by benefics, the person will have good face and eyes.

6. If malefics are in 2 and its lord is with bad planets or is debilitated, the person will have ugly and weak face.
7. If malefics are with the lord of 2 and occupy 12, and malefics aspect the lord of 2, he becomes dumb or will have defective speech.
8. If the lord of 2 is with malefics or in 10 with debilitated Ravi or Ravi and Shani are in 2, he becomes nervous in speech and never commands the respect of the audience.
9. Budha in a quadrant, the lord of 2 is powerful, and Shukra in 5 produce a lover in sublime sciences and a proficient in Astrology.
10. If Kuja is in 2 aspected by Budha or Chandra with Budha in a Kendra, he becomes a great mathematician. If the lord of 2 joins Budha in the quadrants, Guru in birth sign, and Shani in 8 or if Guru occupies one of the quadrants or trines, Shukra is exalted and the lord of 2 is with Budha, the person becomes a clever mathematician.
11. If the lord of 2 is with Guru and Shukra aspected by Ravi and Kuja, and occupies good signs, he becomes a clever logician. If Guru and the lord of 2 are powerful and are aspected by Ravi and Shukra, the person becomes a great grammarian or philologist.
12. If the lord of 2 and Budha are exalted, Shani is in Gopuramsha, or Guru is in Simhasanamsha, or if Guru and Budha occupy quadrants together and Shani is in Parvatamsha, the person becomes a celebrated theologian or religionist.
13. If Guru and Shukra occupy quadrants, the lord of 2 is in Simhasanamsha or Gopuramsha and Budha is in the Navamsha of the lord of birth, he becomes a professor in several branches or Pandit in six Shastras.
14. If the lord of the Navamsha, occupied by Kuja, is in 2 and is powerful and the lord of 2 is in Visheshika, he becomes a wit and humorist. If the lord of 1 is in 2, good planets in 1, or its lord in Parvatamsha, the person will be well versed in the Vedas or religious lore.

15. If the lord of 2 is with the lord of birth aspected by the lord of the birth, Navamsha occupied by the lord of 10, or if the lord of 2 is with the lord of 9 aspected by the lord of the Navamsha occupied by the lord of 1, the man becomes very rich.
16. If the lords of 2 and 9 occupy quadrants aspected by benefics, or if benefics occupy 1, 2, 11 or their lords occupy good houses aspected by the lord of the Navamsha occupied by the lord of 2, the man becomes enormously rich early.
17. If the lord of 1 is in 2, and the lord of 2 is in 11, with the lord 11 in 1, the person becomes rich by hidden treasurers. If the lord of birth is with Guru and occupies a quadrant, and the lord of 2 is in Visheshika, the person acquires much property by self-exertions.
18. If the lord of the Navamsha occupied by the lord of birth joins well with the lord of 2, and occupies quadrants or trines, the person will have much self-acquired property. If the lords of 1, 2 and 11 join together occupying quadrants or trines aspected by benefics, the man will have much wealth in middle life.
19. If the lord of 1, 2 and 3 join together, aspected by male planets or if the lord of 3 is in 2 aspected by or is in conjunction with Kuja, he will have money from brothers.
20. If the lord of birth aspects the lord of 2 occupying quadrants, or good Navamshas, the person earns much by self-exertion.
21. If the lord of 2 is in conjunction with or aspected by the lord of 4, the person gets wealth through the mother.
22. If the lord of 2 is with the lord of 5 and Guru is aspected by the lord of 1, the person gets money through children.
23. If the lord of 7 is with the lord of 2 and is aspected by Shukra, the native gets money through his wife.
24. If the lord of 6 is with the lord of 2 occupying one of the quadrants or trines aspected by benefics, the person gets wealth through enemies.

25. If the lord of 1 is weak, joins with malefics and occupies 12 and the lord of 2 with Ravi is debilitated, the person loses his wealth by fines and confiscations.

26. If the lord of 12 is in 2, the lord of 11 in 12 and the lord of 2 is in 3, 6 or 12, the person loses by fines and penalties.

27. If the lord of 2 and 12 occupy 12 or 2 aspected by the lord of 1, he loses money through king's displeasure.

28. If the lord of 2 and 11 are aspected by Kuja and occupy bad houses or Navamshas, the man loses wealth through king's displeasure, thieves or fire.

29. If the lord of the Navamsha occupied by the lord of 2 is in 3, 6 or 12 with malefics, the person becomes penniless.

30. If the lord of 2, 12 and 11 are unfavourably situated, aspected by or in conjunction with malefics, the man will become a destitute.

31. If the lord of Navamsha occupied by the lord of 12 is with the lord of 2 or is aspected by him, and malefics occupy quadrants, the person becomes very poor.

32. If malefics occupy 2, its lord is in 12 and the lord of 10 is with the lord of 1 or is aspected by him, the person gets into hopeless debt.

33. If the lord of 2 is debilitated or is with Ravi and evil planets occupy 2 and 8, the person will have heavy liabilities.

34. If the lord of 2, 6 and 11 occupy quadrants or trines, the man will be free from debt.

THIRD HOUSE

1. If the lord of 3 and Kuja are in 12 aspected by malefics or if Kuja occupies 3 aspected by evil planets, or if evil planets occupy 3 aspected by malefics or if the lord of 3 is between two bad planets, or if 3 is between two evil planets aspected by or joined with them, without good aspects, the person loses his brothers.

2. If the lord of 3 is debilitated or if 3 is occupied by Shani or aspected by evil planets, or if the 3rd as well as its lord is between evil planets, without good aspects, the persons' brothers die.
3. If the lord of 3 or Kuja occupies 3, 6 or 12 without good aspect, there will be no brothers.
4. If the lord of 3 is with Rahu or Ketu, and occupies unfavourable positions, his brothers die in his early days.
5. If good planets occupy 3 aspected by good planets and its lord is in a good position, the person will have many brothers and they will be successful in life.
6. If the lord of 3 is exalted, Kuja is favourable, aspected by or in conjunction with good planets, his brothers will prosper.
7. If the lord of 3 and Kuja occupy quadrants or trines with good planets, or the lord of 3 is exalted or occupies good Navamsha with good planets, he will have many brothers.
8. If the lord of 3 or Kuja is in an odd sign or Navamsha aspected by Kuja, Guru or Ravi, there will be many brothers.
9. If the lord of 3 or Kuja occupies an even sign, there will be many sisters.
10. If the lord of 3 is in good Navamsha with benefics or Rahu is similarly situated, he will be bold.
11. If the lord of 3 is in 12 and Rahu is not well situated, the person will be courageous in battle.
12. If the lord of 3 is in 12 and Rahu is not well situated, the person will suffer defeat.
13. If the lord of 3 is with Ravi, he becomes courageous; if with Chandra, he becomes bold in mind; if with Kuja, stubborn and angry; if with good planets, thoughtful and calculating.

FOURTH HOUSE

1. If the lord of 4 is with the lord of 1 occupying a good place, or if the lord of 4 occupies one of the trines or quadrants aspected by benefics, or occupies Visheshamsha, the person will own many houses.
2. If the lord of 9 is in a quadrant, the lord of 4 is exalted or well situated, the person will have well furnished houses.
3. If Budha is in 3, the lord of 4 is well placed or if the lord of 4 is with the lord of 10 and Shani occupies a quadrant, the person will own splendid mansion or palaces.
4. If Budha is the lord of 4 aspected by benefits or if Guru is in 4 and its lord is with benefics, there will be respect among relations.
5. If the lord of 4 is with evil planets, or occupies an unfavourable position, he will be neglected by relations. If 4 or its lord is with malefics or aspected by them, the person will have quarrelsome relations.
6. If 4 is movable and its lord is in a similar sign, the person will own many houses in several towns or villages.
7. If the lord of 4 is in 10 and the lord of 10 is in 4 aspected by Kuja, he will have many lands.
8. If benefics occupy 4 and its lord is with benefics, he will have many lands. If the lord of the Navamsha occupied by the lord of 4 occupies a quadrant or is aspected by friendly planets, or is with Kuja or joins him, the person will inherit much landed property from brothers.
9. If the lord of 4 is in 7 and Shukra is in 4 and these are friendly to each other, the person will have much landed property through his wife; if 4 or its lord or Kuja is between two evil planets without any good aspects, the person will inherit much landed property from brothers.
10. If the lord of 4 is in 7 and Shukra in 4 and these are friendly to each other, the person will have much landed property through his wife. If 4 or its lord or Kuja is

between two evil planets without any good aspects, the person will suffer great losses in lands.

11. If the lord of 4 is with powerful Guru and Budha and occupies a quadrant, the person will be very happy and will eat luxuriously.

12. If Shukra or Chandra occupies 4 without any aspect from malefics, the person will eat well and enjoy a jolly life.

13. If malefics occupy 4 without the aspect of benefics, the person will spend a miserable life even when he has much wealth.

14. If the lord of 4 is with Ravi or Kuja without the aspect of good planets and occupies a powerless Navamsha, the person becomes unhappy.

15. If the lord of 4 is debilitated and joins evil planets, the person becomes sinful and licentious.

16. If Chandra and Shukra are in quadrants occupying bad Navamshas, and aspected by or joined with evil planets, the man becomes guilty of undesirable acts with his mother or step-mother.

17. If Chandra is aspected by or joins with evil planets, Ravi occupies a quadrant and the evil planets are in 4 or aspect it, the person becomes guilty of criminal conversation with his mother or mother like relations.

18. If the lord of 4 is joined with or aspected by malefics and the lord of 1 joins with the lord of 7, he will commit sin with aunts — paternal or maternal.

19. If the lord of 7 is in 4 with evil planets and aspected by them, the person will have incestuous relations with sisters.

20. If Shani is in 4 aspected by or joins with malefics, the person will have connection with his sisters.

21. If the lord of 6, Kuja and Chandra occupy 4 aspected by malefics, he will be guilty of immoral conduct with his mother-in-law.

22. If the lord of 4 is with Rahu, strongly aspected by malefics, his mother will be adulterous.

23. If Chandra joins with Rahu or Ketu and is aspected by evil planets, his mother will commit adultery with low men.

24. If Chandra is with Shani aspected by malefics, the mother will have paramours among cultivators. If Chandra is with Budha, mercantile lovers; if Chandra is with Ravi, warrior classes; if with Guru or Shukra, the mother will have priests and religious men as her admirers. Here it is very essential to note that the combination should be powerfully aspected by evil planets, otherwise no adulterous disposition should be ascribed to the mother of the person or to himself or to his sisters or aunts — paternal or maternal. Unless the combination is present as completely as it is described here, and the evil influences are as powerful as they can be, no immorality should be attributed. Virtue is a great problem. Many abstain from fear, from want of opportunities, from timidity, from good company, and from love of good name. Celibacy or chastity, to be really valuable must proceed from a pure love of virtue for its own sake and not from any mercenary or interested motives.

25. If the lord of 1, 4, 9 and 6 join together, the person will be born of adultery.

26. If the lord of 4 is powerful, Chandra joins benefics, and good planets are in 4, the person's mother will live long. If Chandra is exalted, occupies a quadrant, or is with benefics, his mother will live long.

27. If Chandra is between two evil planets, and occupies 6, 8 or 12 and the lord of 4 is debilitated or joins malefics, the child becomes motherless soon.

28. If Shukra is powerful and occupies 4, the person will have gold, clothes, jewels and vehicles. If the lord of 4 is with 8, he will go in palanquins. If Shukra joins with Guru and is in the birth, the person will have many conveyances.

29. If the lord of 9, 1 and 4 occupy 10 or if the lord of 1 and 10 are joined powerfully or if the lord of 9 occupies quadrants or trines, he will have splendid political success.

30. If the lord of 4 is with the lord of 9, aspected by Guru and occupies 1, the person will have a great political advancement.

31. If the lord of 4 is with the lord of 9 and aspects 4, the person becomes a great statesman.

32. If the lord of 9 is in 11, and the lords of 4 and 1 occupy 9, or if the lord of 4 occupies quadrants and the lord of the house occupied by the lord of 4 is with Shukra, the person will have many houses and carriages.

33. If the lord of 4 is in Aries or Scorpio or if Budha is in birth and benefics are in 9, the person will have good position, vehicles, wealth and jewels.

34. If the lord of 2 is exalted, and the lord of 4 is well situated, he becomes an eminent statesman.

35. If 2 is occupied by an exalted planet, or benefics are in quadrants with malefics in 3, 6 and 11, he becomes a king or his equal in power.

36. If the lord of 2 is in birth, lord of 10 in 5 and exalted planets occupy 4, or if the lord of 1, 4 and 9 occupy houses which are quadrants to each other, the person becomes a commander of horses.

37. If exalted planets occupy 10 aspected by the lord of 1 or 9, the person commands a vast army of cavalry.

38. If Shukra is exalted and the lord of 10 is in 1, the person will command many drums.

FIFTH HOUSE

1. If the lord of 5 or the house itself is aspected by powerful Guru, there will be many children.

2. If the lord of 1 joins 5 and its lord is powerful or Guru is well situated, or if the lord of 5 and Guru occupy Visheshamsha, aspected by benefics, the person will have children.

3. If the lord of 2 is in 5, well aspected by Guru or if the lord of birth is with the lord of 5 or aspect each other, the person will have children.
4. If the lords of 1 and 5 occupy quadrants with benefics, and the lord of 2 is powerful or if the lord of the Navamsha occupied by the lord of 5 is with a good planet or is aspected by him, or if the lords of 1 and 9 occupy 7 and the lord of 2 is in 1, the person will have many children.
5. If the lord of 5 is placed between malefics and Guru is in company with malefics, there will be loss of children.
6. If the lords of the Navamshas occupied by the lords of 9, 5, 7 are in conjunction with evil planets, the person will see his children die.
7. If the lord of 5 occupies a debilitated Navamsha or is joined by weak, debilitated or combust planets, aspected by malefics, or occupies with malefics 3, 6 and 12, his children will die.
8. If the lord of 5 occupies one of the evil houses, children will die.
9. If Chandra, Shukra and malefics occupy 10, 7 and 4 respectively with the lord of 1 in conjunction with Budha, or if malefics occupy 12, 5, 8 or if Chandra and Guru occupy birth aspected by Kuja and Shani, the person's family becomes extinct.
10. If all the malefics occupy 4 or if all of them occupy 12, 5, 8 and 1, the person's family becomes extinct.
11. If Budha is the lord of 5 and is with or aspected by benefics, or the lord of 5 is between two benefics, or if Budha is exalted or the lord of 5 is well situated and aspected or Budha occupies 5 or if the lord of the Navamsha occupied by Budha is in a quadrant aspected by benefics, the person becomes very intelligent.
12. If the lord of 5 is between two good planets, Guru is in 5 and Budha is favourable, the person will have penetrating intelligence.

13. If the lord of 1 is debilitated or is with malefics, the person will have no intelligence.

14. If Shani is in 5 or aspects the lord of birth or the lord of the house occupied by Shani is with evil planets, there will be derangement of the brain.

15. If the lord of 5 is aspected by malefics, and 5 is also aspected by them and is placed between two bad planets, the person suffers from heart-disease.

16. If the lord of 5 is in 12 or with its lord and occupies one of the unfavourable houses, there will be heart-disease.

17. If the lord of the Navamsha occupied by the lord of 5 joins with or is aspected by malefics, the person suffers from disease of the heart and will be hard-hearted.

18. If the lord of 5 occupies an unfavourable sign and Budha is in 12 unaspected by malefics, the person suffers from loss of memory.

19. If the lord of 5 is a male, male planet occupies it or a male planet aspects its lord and the Navamsha of 5 is a masculine one, the eldest born will be a male.

20. If the lord of 5 is feminine, the lord is a female and these are aspected by feminine planets, the eldest born will be a female.

21. If the lord of 5 is Shani or Budha and possesses impotent influences or aspects, the child will be eunuch or impotent.

SIXTH HOUSE

1. If the lord of 6 occupies 1 or 8 with evil planets, or if these are not aspected by benefics, the person will have several sores.

2. If the lord of 1, Kuja and Budha occupy 4 or 12, or aspect 6 together, there will be disease in the lower part of the abdomen. If the lord of 6 with Kuja occupies birth, the person will have leprosy or biliousness; if he is with Shani, diseases arising from coldness or numbness; if he is with

Ravi, the person will be passing blood or will suffer complaint from eruption of blood.

3. If the lord of 1 is with the lord of 6 and Ravi, he will have constant fevers; if with Chandra, danger by drowning; if with the Kuja, danger in battle, fights or smallpox; if with Budha, mental disease, or brain fever; if with Shukra danger with wife, if with Shani, flatulence or many complicated diseases; if with Rahu, danger from cobra bites, scorpion stings, thieves, cheats and inexplicable diseases.

4. If the lord of 6 joins with Budha, and Guru occupies birth sign, the sexual organ will be covered with ugly sores and the aspect of evil planets will make it defective or rotten.

5. If the lord of 7 with Shukra occupies 6, the wife becomes barren or will have her sexual organ diseased; if the lord of 6 with the lord of 1 joins with Shani and occupies quadrants or trines the person will be imprisoned or confined; if they join Rahu or Ketu and occupy similar positions, the person will be chained.

6. If Shani occupies 9, Guru in 3, or Ravi in 8 or 12, the man will suffer from amputation of the arms. If Chandra occupies 6 and Kuja and Guru are in 8, the man will have his feet cut off.

7. If Shani occupies 1, Rahu is in 7, Shukra is in 10, he will have his head cut off. If weak Chandra is aspected by Rahu and Shani occupies 1, the person will have his head smashed or broken.

8. If Chandra is in 6, 8 or 12 and has the aspect of the lord of 4 or if Shani is debilitated and occupies an unfavourable Navamsha, aspected by evil planets, the person will die by accident.

9. If the lord of 6 and 8 or Kuja joins with the lord of 3 and occupy bad signs or Navamsha, or if Ravi and Kuja aspect each other or occupy their mutual Navamshas, the person will die in battle.

10. If Chandra is in 6 with Kuja, the person will suffer from brain disease or jaundice; if Chandra is in 6 with Shani and Ravi he will have his death from serpents or pains in stomach.

11. If Kuja and Budha occupy 6 aspected by Shukra and Chandra and occupy unfavourable Navamshas, there will be consumption.

12. If 6 is occupied by Shani and Kuja aspected by Ravi and Rahu and the lord of the birth is weak, the person will be constantly sick.

13. If 6 is occupied by Shani and Gulika aspected by Ravi, Kuja and Rahu without good aspects, he suffers from gout or asthma.

14. If Chandra is in a watery sign and the lord of that sign occupies 6, the man suffers incurable venereal diseases and stone in the bladder. If Chandra is in 6, Shani in 8, evil planets in 12 and the lord of the birth is in an unfavourable Navamsha, the person will suffer from complicated nasal disease.

15. If the lord of 6 occupies a Kendra aspected by malefics and they also occupy 6 or if the lord of 6 is in birth and the lord of birth is in 6 with Shani or Gulika, or if the lord of 6 is with evil planets, or is placed between them, or is aspected by malefics, the person will suffer much from enemies and their machinations.

16. If the lord of 6 is in 3 or 12 and is debilitated or is in a bad sign and the lord of 1 is well situated, the person will become foeless.

17. If 6 or its lord is aspected by or joined with benefics, the person gains over his enemies and thereby benefits himself.

18. If the lord of 6 or the lord of birth is weak and is seen by benefics, the person gains over his enemies.

19. If the lord of 1 occupies 6 or aspects him, the person suffers much from his cousins. If Guru and Shukra are

in 1, with the lord of 6 to be aspected by Shani, Kuja or Rahu, the man suffers much from the intrigues of his cousins.

20. If the lord of 9 occupies 6 or is aspected by its lord of the latter and is with Shani or Kuja, the person will suffer from thieves, fires and vagabonds.

21. If 6 is with benefics or its lord is with them or has their aspect, or if he is between two evil planets, the person will be fond of pulses and pickles.

22. If Shukra and Budha are in 6 combined with or aspected by benefics and occupy good Navamsha, the person will be fond of sweets. If Budha joins Shukra or is seen by malefics he will be fond of sour or pungent things.

SEVENTH HOUSE

1. If Shukra is in 7, the person becomes passionate; if Budha is there, he will be fond of other family women; if Guru is there, he will be fond of his own wife; if Shani, fond of ugly women; if Kuja, fond of many women; if Ravi, he will illtreat his wife.

2. If the lord of 2, 7 and 6 occupy birth, and Shukra is with malefics, the person will have many wives.

3. If evil planets occupy 1 and 6, the person will be licentious. If the lords of 1, 6 and 2 join malefics or occupy 7, or Shani is with the lord of 7 or is aspected by evil planets, the person becomes very immoral.

4. If the lord of 7 is with Rahu or Ketu aspected by malefics or if the lord of 10, 2 and 7 occupy 10, the person becomes very adulterous. If 4 is occupied by even one planet, or if the lord of 5 is aspected by the lord of 7 or 6, the person becomes fond of other women.

5. If weak Chandra is in 7 with malefics, or if evil planets occupy 7 with its lord, the person becomes fond of others' wives.

6. If the lord of 5 is in 7 and the lord of 7 is with malefics, and Shukra is weak, the wife dies during pregnancy.

7. If the lord of 2 as well as the lord of 7 occupy their own houses, the person will have only one wife.
8. If the lord of 7 is powerful, exalted or retrograde and occupies 1, the person will have many wives.
9. If the lord of 1 is in 12, evil planets occupy 7 and the lord of 2 is in conjunction with malefics, the person will have two wives.
10. If the lord of 7 is with good planets and is unfavourably situated, and evil planets are in 7, the person will have two marriages.
11. If many evil planets occupy 2 or 7, or their lords are aspected by them, the person will marry thrice. If the lord of birth occupies 10 with strong Budha, and the lord of 7 with Chandra in 3, the person becomes a women hunter.
12. If the lords of 12 and 2 occupy 3, aspected by Guru or the lord of 9, the person will be surrounded by women.
13. If the lord of 7 occupies one of the quadrants or trines, or occupies good houses or Navamsha or joins with the lord of 10, the man will have numberless women.
14. If the lords of 7 and 11 join together or aspect each other or powerfully occupy trines, he will have many women.
15. If the lord of 9 is in 7 and its lord is in 4 or the lords of 7 and 11 occupy quadrants, the person will marry many women.
16. If the lord of the sign occupied by the Navamsha joined by the lord of 7 is with Budha or good planets, and occupies Parvatamsha, or is otherwise powerful, the person will marry a hundred women.
17. Take the lord of the Navamsha occupied by Shukra and then find out the lord of the sign occupied by him and if the latter occupies a quadrant or Gopuramsha, the person will have 300 wives.
18. If an evil planet is with the lord of 7 and another occupies 7 and the lord of the Navamsha occupied by the lord of 7

happens to be an evil planet, the person gets a miserable wife.

19. If the lord of 7 occupies a bad place and Shukra is weak, the person will have a bad wife.

20. If the lord 7 and Shukra are debilitated, and not aspected by benefics, the person will have a wretched wife.

21. If a good planet is with the lord of 7 and another occupies it, and both are aspected by benefics, the person will have a desirable wife.

22. If the lord of 7, Shukra and the lord of 10 occupy good Navamshas, or otherwise powerful, or if Shukra is exalted or occupies a good Navamsha or if the lord of 7 is with Guru, or is seen by him or joins good Navamshas, or if the lord of 7 is aspected by Ravi with Shukra and Guru occupies 7, the person will have an excellent, loving and chaste wife. His home will be a paradise on earth.

23. If Ravi and the lord of 7 are powerful, in conjunction with the benefics or occupy good Navamshas, the spouse will be faithful.

24. If Chandra and the lord of 7 are in bad places and are aspected by or joined with malefics, or placed between them, the wife becomes unfaithful.

25. If Shukra and the lord of 7 in company with debilitated planets are in debilitated houses, and occupy evil Navamshas, the person will have a cruel, adulterous and murderous wife.

26. If Rahu or Ketu joins the lord of 7, not aspected by benefics and occupies unfavourable houses, the person will have a wife who administers poison or adopts other means to kill him, and she will be licentious and careless of reputation.

27. If the lord of 7 is close to the lord of 1, or if 1, 2 and 7 are occupied by good planets or their lords join good Navamshas, or have the aspect of benefics, there will be early marriage.

28. If the lord of 7 with an evil planet and occupies trines, Shukra is with malefics and the lord of 2 is in 10, there will be late marriage.

29. If Ravi is in 7, there will be intercourse with barren women; if Chandra is in 7, with maids and servile classes; if Kuja is in 7, with women in menses; if Budha, with mercantile, barren and poor women; if Guru, with priestly and religious women; if Shukra, with pregnant women, if Shani, with old or immatured girls.

30. If the above planets occupy 4, he will be guilty of the same offences and the places of adultery are thus determined. For Ravi, the places is garden or forest; for Chandra, in houses; for Kuja, near walls or dilapidated buildings; for Budha, pleasure walks or places of resort; for Guru, in temples or holy places; for Shukra, in watery places; for Shani or Rahu or Ketu, instable sheds, garages or other places where animals and vehicles are kept.

31. If all the quadrants are occupied by evil planets,. without being aspected by or in company with benefics, he will have intercourse with animals.

32. If all the quadrants are aspected by malefics, the person will have connection with beasts.

33. If evil planets occupy quadrants or if Shani joins Gulika, the person enjoys women like a brute.

34. If Ravi is with Shani and Kuja occupies 4, or if Rahu occupies 7 and Kuja is in 4, the person enjoys sexual intercourse like a brute.

35. If Shani is seen by Shukra or occupies Aries or Scorpio with Shukra or joins with the lord of 2, the person will be madly fond of sexual organs and will kiss or fondle them, or will be guilty of solitary sin.

36. If the lord of 10 is seen by Shani or occupies Aries of Scorpio, aspected by or is in conjunction with Shukra, the person will kiss the sexual organs or make much of them. If the lord of 1 is debilitated or similarly aspected, he will be guilty of similar indiscretions.

37. If Kuja occupies 7, the wife's breast will be dried up, if Rahu or Shani is in 7, she will have hanging or ugly chest; if Ravi, she will have erect and strong breast; if Budha, Shukra, Guru or full Chandra, she will have developed and attractive breast.

38. If the lord of 7 is with benefics or with watery planets, or occupies watery signs aspected by Guru, the person will have a wife with a luxuriantly developed chest. If Ravi or Kuja is with Shani or Gulika, and the lord of 7 occupies an evil division, his wife will have a long sexual organ.

39. If the lord of 7 is with Guru, and occupies a good division, her sexual organ will be moderate, and if evil planets join with him, the organ will be very long.

40. If the lord of 7 is in a watery sign, and 7 is a watery sign, aspected by full Chandra or if Chandra occupies 7, aspected by Shukra, the sexual organ of the wife will be soft and secreting.

41. If full Chandra is in 7 or a watery Navamsha aspected by Guru, the sexual organ will be soft and tender.

42. If Shukra is exalted or occupies a watery Navamsha and joins with Ravi, the wife will have little inclination for sexual intercourse.

43. If 7 is owned by an evil planet, its lord is between two malefics, or joins, or is aspected by them, the sexual organ of the wife will be hard, and she will require strong intercourse.

44. If the lord of 7 is weak, occupies a bad house or joins with powerless planets, the wife will have her organ dry and she will require good sexual operation.

EIGHTH HOUSE

1. If there are many malefics in 8, the private parts will be diseased; if good planets aspect them, there will be much relief.

2. If the lord of 8 is with malefics or is aspected by them, or is between them, or occupies bad houses, or in 8, the person will be disgraced.
3. If 8 becomes a movable sign and its lord is also in a movable sign, the person will die in a foreign country.
4. If 8 and its lord are in a fixed sign and Shani is similarly placed, the person will die in his own home, and if the above three are in common signs, the person will die while travelling.

NINTH HOUSE

1. If the lord of 9 is in 8, or in movable sign, the child will be born when its father is not in the place.
2. If Chandra is in 9 with malefics or Shukra, or if its lord is with them, the person will have criminal connection with his teachers' wives.
3. If the lord of Navamsha occupied by the lord of 9 is with evil planets, or if Chandra occupies 9 with malefics, the person commits indecent act with elderly matrons.
4. If Chandra is weak or occupies an evil Navamsha, or Shukra is similarly situated, or if the lord of 9 is debilitated or occupies a bad Navamsha with Shukra, the person has connection with motherly relations.
5. If Guru or Shukra is exalted or occupies favourable division, and the lord of 1 is powerful, the person becomes charitable, honest and straightforward.
6. If the lord of 9 occupies the Navamsha of Guru or Budha aspected by benefics, or is placed between them, he will be a man of principles.
7. If good planets occupy 9 and its lord occupies a weak Navamsha or unfavourable division, the person does charity with a view to become famous.
8. If Rahu and Shani are in 9 and its lord is aspected by Gulika in the Navamsha, the person becomes cruel-hearted and impious.

9. If the lord of 9 is a good planet, and Ravi is in conjunction with a good planet, the person will have paternal bliss.
10. If the lords of 1 and 9 are powerful as well as Ravi and aspected by benefics, the person will be obedient to his father.
11. If the lord of 9 is in one of the quadrants or trines aspected by, or is in conjunction with good planets the person becomes wealthy.
12. If the lord of 2 is in 9 and the lord of 9 is in 11 and the lord of 11 is in 2 aspected by or in conjunction with the lord of 10, the person becomes extremely wealthy.
13. If the lord of 9 joins with the lord of 3 aspected by, or is in conjunction with benefics, and occupies good Navamshas, the person gets much wealth from his brothers.
14. If the lord of 9 is in 10 aspected by powerless or debilitated planets and occupies bad divisions or if the lord of 9 is weak, malefics are in 9 and the lord of 1 is bad, the person becomes poor.
15. If the lord of 1 occupies 9 and the lord of 9 joins 1, or if the lord of 9 occupies 11, or if the lords of 11 and 9 join together and are in 2, the man gets rich again. Here, it is meant that the man first gets money, loses it and gets it back again. He has ups and downs in his life.
16. If the lord of 10 is in 9 and the lord of 9 is powerful and is aspected by Shukra or Guru, the person becomes very religious.
17. If the lord of 9 is exalted, and is aspected by good planets, and benefics are in 9, or if the lord of 1 is seen by the lord of 9 and they occupy quadrants or trines, the person becomes very charitable.
18. If the lord of 9 is in 4, and the lord of 10 occupies quadrants, and the lord of 12 has the aspect of Guru, the man will be charitable.

19. If the lord of 5 joins 9 and the lord of 9 occupies 10 aspected by the lord of 10, the person receives liberal gifts or charities.

20. If the lord of 9 is seen by the lord of 10 and occupies quadrants or trines, the person receives very substantial charitable gifts.

TENTH HOUSE

1. If the lord of 10, 2 and Budha are powerful, he will perform sacrifice. If Shukra, Budha and Guru occupy 3, 6 and 12, the person becomes irreligious. If Rahu or Shani is in 10, he bathes in holy rivers.
2. If Budha is in 12 or the lord of 12 is exalted, or if Chandra occupies 3 being watery sign aspected by benefics, the person will bathe in sacred rivers.
3. If Guru joins Budha or Kuja, the person builds temples, mantapas and choultries.
4. If the lord of 10 is in it, the person repairs old buildings, temples, churches, or if the lord of 1 occupies Gopuramsha, he repairs tanks and wells.
5. If Budha is in 10 and its lord is in 9 without malefics, the person performs many sacrifices.
6. If the lord of 10 is Budha and aspected by benefics or is in good Navamsha, the person commands good respect.
7. If Ravi is in 10 with Kuja and if the lord of 10 occupies any one of the quadrants, the person will be cruel and greatly feared.
8. If the lord of 10 is with Shani as also the lord of 8, and joins cruel Navamsha or quadrants, the person will give cruel and unreasonable commands and he will be greatly feared.
9. If Ravi and Shani are in 10, or the lord of 10 is between evil planets, the man becomes very unpopular.
10. If 10 is occupied by good planets, or its lord is well situated and aspected by benefics, the person will be popular, persevering and steady in carrying out his works.

11. If malefics occupy 10 and its lord is similarly joined by them, the person becomes careless of his reputation.

12. If the lord of 6 is in 10 and the lord of 10 is with Shani and occupies quadrants or trines, the person commands many servants of both sexes.

13. If the lord of 10 or the house itself is seen by benefics in company with Shani, the person will command many servants.

14. If malefics occupy 10 without being aspected by or in conjunction with good planets, the person will have weakness.

ELEVENTH HOUSE

1. If the lord of 11 occupies one of the quadrants or trines or 11 is with malefics or if the lord of 2 occupies 11 and the lord of 11 occupies 2 or these two occupy quadrants, the person will be very wealthy.

2. If 11 or its lord is placed between two good planets, or occupies good divisions, or if the lord of the house occupied by the lord of 11 is seen by benefics or placed between them, the person will be rich.

3. If the lord of the Navamshas occupied by the lord of 11 is powerful and is aspected by the lord of 2, he will be very rich.

4. If the lord of the Thrimshamsha occupied by the lord of 11 becomes powerful by being in company with benefics, and aspected by the lord of 10, the person becomes wealthy.

5. If the above lords are in conjunction with malefics, the man loses money.

6. The direction in which a person gets wealth will be determined by the sign occupied by the lord of 11 or that indicated by the house itself.

7. If the lord of 11 is a good planet aspected by benefics, the person will have good ears.

8. If the above planets are not powerful and have bad associations, the person will have bad ears, and if the planets are debilitated or combust, the person becomes deaf.
9. If 11 is occupied by benefics, and its lord is well situated, the person will have elder brothers and they will be successful, and their sexes must be determined by the planets and the signs they occupy.
10. If the lord of 11 and those who are in it are powerful and occupy good divisions, the person will have powerful friends, but if they are weak, the person will have cheating and false companions.

TWELFTH HOUSE

1. If 12 is with malefics, as well as its lord, and both have evil aspect, or if 12 or its lord is with Shani and Gulika, and occupies bad places, the person will waste his money for immoral and illegal purposes.
2. If the lord of 12 is aspected by the lord of 7 and these two are powerless, his money will be wasted through his wife's influence.
3. If the lord of 12 is in one of the trines, evil planets aspect quadrants, and if they occupy bad divisions, or if the lord of 12 is aspected by benefics, or if the lord of 10 and occupies good Navamshas, the person spends his money on charitable purposes.
4. If the lord of 12 is weak and is seen by the lord of 6 in conjunction with malefics or Gulika, money will be spent on account of enemies.
5. If the lord of 5 is weak or joins evil planets, and aspects the lord of 12, the person loses money through children.
6. If evil planets occupy 12 or its lord is aspected by or is in company with weak planets, the person suffers from bodily weakness or defect.
7. If Rahu and Gulika occupy 12 and are aspected by the lord of 6 or if the lord of 12 occupies bad divisions or

joins with evil planets without good planets, the person will go to hell.

8. If exalted planets occupy 12, and are aspected by good planets, and occupy Devalokamsha or such good divisions, the person goes to heaven.
9. If benefics occupy 12 or its lord joins with them, the person will be fond of good furniture.
10. If the lord of 12 is exalted, joins good division and is aspected by benefics, the person will have nice cots and costly curtains.
11. If the lord of 12 is exalted and is aspected by the lord of 9, the person will have gilt or highly ornamental furniture.

KIND OF WORSHIP

1. If Shukra occupies 5 with conjunction or these together aspect 5, the person will be fond of worshipping Goddesses.
2. If male planets join or aspect 5, the person will worship gods.
3. If Shani is in 5, or sees that sign, the person will be fond of holding communication with devils, spirits and hobgoblins.
4. If Chandra occupies or aspects 5, the person will be clever in magic or such tricks.

THE RESULTS OF THE BHAVAS

The results of the twelve Bhavas have now been given at considerable length. A 'Bhava' in Sanskrit means a house of division of the Zodiac which signifies a series of events, connected with human existence. Results detailed in this Chapter, by the combinations of planets, must be carefully calculated and then predicted. When two or more planets combine, in certain positions, to produce a definite result it must be predicted in full only when they are equally strong and placed in the exact relationship mentioned by the astrological formulas. But if one of the planets is strong, and another is weak, then the result will be considerably modified, and if the astrologer through ignorance of the sources of strength and weakness of the planets, predicts results sketched above for that combination, he will have more chances of failure than success.

I shall illustrate what I mean. For instance, certain combinations of planets are supposed to give a person 'hidden treasure.' This is a combination which enables a man to become suddenly rich, without many of the worries, to which a man will be subjected, when he tries to earn money honestly. It will be, therefore, tempting for a man to consult an astrologer and have a false assurance from him, that he would suddenly come by hidden treasure. The quantity of treasure thus procured may vary from a few rupees to a very large sum. The combination is thus stated. "If the lord of 1st is in the 2nd and the lord of the 2nd is in the 11th and the lord of the 11th is in the 1st, the person comes by hidden treasure". Suppose Mesha is Lagna, its lord is Kuja and he must be in the 11th or Kumbha. The lord of Kumbha is, Shani and he must be in the 1st or Mesha. This is one combination which gives treasure trove.

Take another example. Vrishabha is Lagna. Its lord is Shukra and he must be in the 2nd or Mithuna. The lord of Mithuna is Budha, and he must be in the 11th or Meena. The lord of Meena is Guru and must be in the 1st or Lagna.

The 1st example has Kuja where Shukra and Shani are enemies. In the second example, Shukra, Budha and Guru are also enemies. But there is a difference. The lord of Lagna in the 1st will be Kuja, and he is an inveterate enemy of Shukra and Shani. The lord of Vrishabha is Shukra and he is a great friend to Budha, but he is unfriendly to Guru. If these combinations are produced before me, I would at once predict, for these reasons that one born in Vrishabha with this combination, will get a better 'find' than one who is born in Mesha. Besides, Shukra is the Karaka (lord) of treasure trove or Nidhi and Nikshepa and this greatly adds value to the strength of the combination. Take Vrischika, the lord of it is Kuja and he must be in the 2nd of Dhanus. Guru is his friend and he must be in Vrischika. Here the friction between the planets is less and the person gets a better 'find'.

Similarly, the sources of the strength of the houses or Bhavas, their situation between good or evil planets, the strength of their lords, their aspects, situation and conjunction; and the good or evil divisions where all these occupy in the Shadvargas must be taken into careful consideration. Exaltations and debilitations, friendly or unfriendly houses, malefic and benefic aspects, and the various sources of strength, positional, directional, lateral, temporal and Naisargica must also be taken into consideration, before the results can be safely predicted. **"To dive into the future is no easy job, and one must be well up in all these details."** Otherwise he will be in the same sorry position, that a mathematician would be, who neglects his account of ciphers, and only tries to take note of the figures. Sciences are generally difficult to understand and require a special knack, great devotion and higher intelligence to master them, but Astrology is the grandest of the known sciences and the intellect, which tries to grasp its difficult problems, must have commensurate capacity to do justice to it, if it really wants to produce satisfaction to itself and to those who come for consultation. Astrology is a huge chemical science where the details of composition and decomposition must be carefully analysed, the effects are expressed in a symbolical language, which can be easily mastered by good concentration of the mind.

❖❖❖

CHAPTER - 12

MISCELLANEOUS COMBINATIONS

The following combinations are briefly sketched here so that the reader might see, that even when the previously stated conjunctions are not present, the person may, shall be in good or bad condition, and that the astrologer has to account for it by examining whether any one of the undermentioned combinations is found in the horoscope. These are permanent combinations and they affect the party more or less with their main influences, all through his life, subject, of course, to such special modifications as are brought about by the planetary periods or Dashas.

1. **Rajju**: If all the planets occupy movable signs, it is called, Rajju, and the person will be jealous of others success, living in foreign territory, fond of travelling, and capable of enduring much fatigue.

2. **Musala**: If all the planets are in fixed signs, he will be fond of good name, conceited, wealthy and capable of undertaking and managing several works single handed.

3. **Nala**: If all the planets are in common signs, the person will be persevering, wealthy and very skilful in all the arts.

4. If Chandra occupies a quadrant from Ravi, the person will be impolite, poor, ignorant, unskilful and miserable.

5. If Guru occupies Panaparas from Ravi, the person will be moderately intelligent, well-to-do and ordinary in his occupation.

6. If Chandra occupies Apoklimas from Ravi, the person will be very polite, extremely wealthy, highly intelligent, well-educated, and very skilful in arts and sciences.

7. **Adhiyoga**: When Guru, Shukra, and Budha are in 6, 7 and 8 from Chandra, it is called Adhiyoga. Here all the planets might occupy any one of these house, or two together in one house, or three, one in each house then

he will be a king, minister or commander-in-chief, according to their power.

Results: Great wealth, happiness, universal conquest, loss to enemies, long life and excellent health. If evil planets occupy the above houses, the person will become a tyrant, but still will enjoy the same advantages and becomes a bad, but a great man. Many authors are of opinion that Adhiyoga exists only when the benefics occupy the 6th, 7th and 8th houses from the Moon. Bhattotpala, learned commentator of Varaha Mihira's works, also recognises Papadhiyoga.

8. **Shunapha**: Planets (excepting Ravi) occupying the 2nd house from Chandra — the person will become a king or his equal, wealthy, self-exerting, well-educated, intelligent, and will have good reputation.
9. **Anapha**: Planets in the 12th house from Chandra save Ravi — the person will have majestic appearance, good health, polite manners, tact, fame, equanimity of mind, enjoyment of all sexual pleasures, fine taste, good jewels, furniture, sweet scents, with a nature that brooks no opposition.
10. **Dhuradhura**: Planets in 2 and 12 from Chandra excepting Ravi—enjoys all kinds of worldly enjoyments, excellent conveyances, immense wealth, good and generous disposition, obedient servants and high political power.
11. **Kemadruma**: No planets in the 2nd and the 12th houses from Chandra—dirty, indolent, careless of character, bodily and mental disease, fond of mean and undignifying acts, poor, cruel, a hanger on others, devoid of feelings of self respect. The person will have these even when he is born in a royal family, much more so, of course, when this combination is present in other horoscopes if Chandra is with any planet or any one of the planets occupies quadrants from Chandra, the evil results above sketched will be considerably mitigated, but occasionally the person will feel them. In these cases the presence or absence of Ravi will make no difference.

If Kuja causes any one of these Yogas, he will produce great elevation of spirits, courage, wealth and romantic nature. If Budha causes it, the person becomes clever, eloquent, and highly versed in all arts and sciences. If Guru causes it, he will be wealthy, charitable, happy and highly respected by rulers. If Shukra, he will be licentious and enjoys different sexual pleasures. If Shani, he will enjoy comforts at the cost of others, popular leader of castemen.

12. **Vasumathiyoga**: If 3, 6, 10 and 11 from birth or Chandra are occupied by Shukra, Guru and Budha, the person will become a millionaire or extremely wealthy. If two planets, moderate, if one planet, ordinary.
13. If benefics occupy quadrants or trines and malefics are in 3, 6 and 11, he will become a statesman.
14. If Guru and Budha join together, or aspect each other, the person will have immense political power or influence.
15. **Neecha Bhanga Rajayoga**: If the lord of the house, where a planet chances to be, debilitated, or the planet which will have its exaltation there, occupies any one of the quadrants from Chandra, the person will rise from poverty to eminence.
16. **Raja Mudradhikara Yoga**: If Chandra occupies any one of the quadrants and is aspected by powerful Guru or Shukra, the person will become a great magistrate.
17. If debilitated planets occupy their exalted Navamshas or if the exalted planets occupy their debilitated Navamshas, the person will become an eminent citizen.
18. If the 12 zodiacal signs are equally divided into 3 parts, we get 4 signs for each division. Divide the life of the person into 3 equal periods. If the first four houses from birth contain 'the largest number of benefics, the person generally enjoys fortune in the first one-third period of his life.' If the second division contains the largest number of benefics, then he will have best fortune in the second one-third period of his life, the last division contains the

largest number of benefics, then he will have the best fortune in the third or last part of his life. If they are equally distributed then he will have continuous fortune. This will enable students to predict miseries, dismissals, prosecutions, losses of wealth and sorrow or happiness in the different periods of a man's life. In fact, the ups and downs in life are to be judged roughly by this clue.

19. If Guru is in 1, Budha is in quadrants aspected by the lords of 1 or 9, then he will attain a great position.
20. If Guru is in 5, 7 or 9 aspected by the lord of birth, the person will flourish in politics.
21. If Shani is in one of the quadrants, trines or Moolathrikona or is exalted or aspected by the lord of 10, the person will become a statesman.
22. If the lord of 10 is in 8 or is exalted or is in friendly Navamsha, and occupies Parvatamsha, he will become a great officer.
23. If Guru is in 5 and Chandra is in one of the quadrants from Guru and the lord of the house occupied by Chandra is in a fixed sign, the person will become an eminent statesman.
24. If the lord of the Navamsha occupied by Chandra is in quadrants, or trines, or occupies any of the quadrants from Budha, the man will become a great lord.
25. If Guru with Kuja is in 2 or 3, and Rahu is in 5, the person will become a great lord.
26. If the lord of the Navamsha occupied by the lord of 9 joins 5 or 4, the person will become a great statesman.
27. If Shani and Rahu occupy 10 aspected by the lord of 9 and the lord of the birth is with an evil planet, he will become an eminent officer.
28. If Shani is in birth without favourable aspect and other planets are debilitated or occupy bad divisions, he will become a beggar and will ruin his family.

29. If the lord of the birth occupies 12, evil planets are in 10 and Chandra is with Kuja, the person will go for begging with a loathsome body, suffer all the pangs of misery and will be hated by all.
30. If Shani is in quadrants, Chandra in 1 and Guru in 12, the person will get worthless children and wife, and becomes a miserable wretch.
31. If Shukra is debilitated and is in the Navamsha of Shani, Ravi and Chandra occupy 12 and Shani aspects 7, the person will depend upon others for livelihood and will lead a worthless life.
32. If malefics are in 4 and 5 and Chandra is in 12 or 8, the man will become blind.
33. If Chandra occupies 10, Budha in 7 and Shani in 2, he will have defective organs or will lose some of them by disease.
34. If weak Chandra is in 4 aspected by malefics alone, the person will have falls from his coaches or horses.
35. If Chandra and Ravi occupy 9 without good aspects, the father will be drowned.
36. If Ravi and Chandra are in Pisces, aspected by malefics, the father will be drowned.
37. If Guru is debilitated as well as Ravi, with evil planets in quadrants, the person will be guilty of infanticide.
38. If malefics occupy quadrants and Shukra is in 8, the person will be a great hunter.
39. If Chandra and Budha are in 10 aspected by Ravi in conjunction with malefics and join inauspicious Amshas, the person will kill birds daily.
40. If Chandra is in 12 or 7 with Shukra, the person will lose his left eye.
41. If Ravi is in 5, 8, or 9, the person will have his body pierced through.

42. **Gadayoga**: All planets occupying the two nearest quadrants as in 1 and 4 or 4 and 10 or 10 and 1 compose this yoga, then the person will be fond of religious rites, wealthy, clever in earning money.

43. **Shakata**: All planets in 1 and 7, then the person will live by carriage or hiring coaches.

44. **Vihaga**: All planets in 4 and 10, then the person will be a messenger, vagrant and quarrelsome.

45. **Hala**: All the planets in trines to each other with none in birth sign, the person will live entirely by cultivation.

46. **Shrungataka**: All the planets in 1, 5 and 9, the person will live happily in old age.

47. **Yoopa**: All the planets in 1, 2, 3 and 4, then the person will be charitable, sincere and fond of sacrificial rites.

48. **Ishu**: All the planets in 4, 5, 6 and 7, then the person will be an executioner, master of a prison or jail maker of arrows bows.

49. **Shaktha**: All the planets in 7, 8, 9 and 10, then the person will be lazy, unhappy, poor and miserable.

50. **Danda**: All planets in 10, 11, 12 and 1 then the person would be neglected by close relations.

51. **Koota**: All planets in 4, 5, 6, 7, 8, 9 and 10 in a line, then the person will be a terrible liar, miserly, official-in-charge of jail birds.

52. **Chandra**: All planets in 7, 8, 9, 10, 11 and 12 in a line, then the person will help his friends and relations and enjoy his old life.

53. **Dhanus**: All planets in 10, 11, 12, 1, 2, 3 and 4 in a line, the person will be a warrior.

54. **Ardhachandra**: All planets in 7 houses in a regular line wherever they might commence from, then the person will be popular, handsome and a great minister or secretary to government.

55. **Valaki**: All planets in 7 houses in any manner or order, then the person will be keen-sighted, fond of dancing and singing.

56. **Damini**: All planets in 6 houses in any order, then the person will be liberal, fond of helping others, will have many cattle.

57. **Pasha**: All planets in 5 houses, then the person will be honest and just in the acquisition of wealth, possesses faithful servants and devoted friends.

58. **Kedara**: All planets in 4 houses then the person will be a successful cultivator, fond of helping his fellow-creatures.

59. **Shoola**: All planets in 3 houses, then the person will be a warrior, avaricious, fond of murdering or butchering, spiller of human blood.

60. **Yuga**: All planets in two houses, the person will be poor, filthy, atheist and miserable.

61. **Golaka**: All planets in one house, the person will be poor, ignorant, lazy, going against the world, servant in carrying communications from place to place.

I have stated at considerable length some of the miscellaneous combinations which are interesting and instructive. In making predictions, readers have to bear in mind the fact that while a man has, what may be called general happiness, he may also be subjected to petty local or domestic afflictions and inconveniences. No one can be said to be perfect in the enjoyment of worldly bliss. The rich man has his own cares, while the poor man often enjoys happiness, and the ingredients which go to make men happy or miserable depend upon various considerations. The construction and the attitude of mind towards its surroundings, plays an important part in producing happiness or misery.

When some combinations are predicting good, others act against them, and the astrologer will have to see which influences are strong and effective and which are not so.

Without a careful study of the earlier part of this book, the subsequent portions will not be intelligible. A gentleman of ordinary abilities can master the details in less than a month. All combinations are subject to influences of the planetary periods or Dashas, as the general law is subject to be varied by the local or special law, and the position, therefore, of the planet whose Dasha commences becomes very important and effects the general results, a great deal. Then again the continuous movements of the planets, called Gochara should not be forgotten in judging of any horoscopes. Deep study, intelligent instruction from competent scholars in the science, good memory, much experience, and careful judgement are the keys with which the locked doors into the futurity or humanity can be opened.

A student who only reads the book for the first time, and finds the results unsatisfactory, will be like a man, who is anxious to learn the art of swimming, but who neglects the ordinary precaution to ensure success therein. The result of hastiness in the sentence of astrological predictions will lead to confusion and contradiction, while the results of hastiness and indiscretion in swimming will lead to drowning of the person, perhaps never to rise again. Patience and devotion above will overcome all obstacles.

In Golaka, it is necessary to have all the planets in one house. The question arises whether that is possible when Rahu and Ketu are taken. These planets (Shadowy) are always 180° apart and therefore can never meet. But in all the older astrological works they are not taken note of and the authors refer only to the seven other planets. It is possible to see that all the seven planets meet in one house perhaps at very long intervals. In the beginning of the present creation of the world it is alleged by experts, that all the planets were started with different velocities from the first house or Aries, and when all of them meet in that house again, there will be a 'Pralaya' or general destruction.

❖❖❖

CHAPTER - 13

STELLAR EFFECTS OR INFLUENCES OF NAKSHATRAS

I shall first give the effects of the 27 constellations at the time of birth, and then the influences of the Moon when he moves in them.

1. **Aswini**: Polite, sweet speech, fond of jewels, good dress, handsome, popular, intelligent, expert in arts and sciences.
2. **Bharani**: Truthful, persevering, healthy, skilful, free from cares and happy.
3. **Krittika**: Voracious eater, fond of others wives, handsome and famous.
4. **Rohini**: Truthful, man of principles, polite, steady, and handsome.
5. **Mrigasira**: Capricious, skilful, cowardly, talkative, light-hearted, rich and fond of enjoyment.
6. **Arudra**: Dissimulator, proud, ungrateful, cruel-hearted, sinful and fond of killing.
7. **Punarvasu**: Penitent, happy, good tempered, little cracked, sickly, thirsty, contented with small gains.
8. **Pushya**: Very quiet, popular, learned, wealthy and fond of good deeds.
9. **Aslesha**: Pretender, cheating partners, sinful, ungrateful and clever in swindling others.
10. **Makha**: Enjoyment in life, many servants, great wealth, religious, respectful, highly contented.
11. **Uttaraphalguni**: Good speech, liberal, handsome, traveller and submissive.
12. **Poorvaphalguni**: Popular, learned, enjoyable life and free from cares.
13. **Hasta**: Hopeful, steady, given to strong liquors, unkind and pilferer.

14. **Chitra**: Charming eyes and fond of various coloured clothes.
15. **Swati**: Polite, moral, merchant, kind-hearted, sweet words and fond of doing meritorious deeds.
16. **Visakha**: Narrow-minded, jealous, miser, good-looking, clever in the art of speech and quarrelsome.
17. **Anuradha**: Wealthy, residence in a foreign country, not capable of enduring hunger and roving habits.
18. **Jyeshta**: Jolly, few friends, charitable and unreasonably angry.
19. **Moola**: Conceited, wealthy, happy kind-hearted, resolute and enjoyment in life.
20. **Poorvashada**: Good and agreeable wife, conceited and constant in friendship.
21. **Uttarashada**: Polite, charitable, grateful, popular and many friends.
22. **Sravana**: Rich, learned, good and chaste wife, enjoyable life and famous.
23. **Dhanishta**: Wealthy, liberal, courageous, fond of music and avaricious.
24. **Satabisha**: Eloquent and distinct speaker, gambler, fond of bad women, murder of enemies, adventurous and deep-hearted.
25. **Poorvabhadra**: Sorrowful, submissive to women, wealthy, clever and miserly.
26. **Uttarabhadra**: Eloquent speaker, happy, blessed with children and grandchildren, unrivalled and charitable.
27. **Revati**: Well-developed body, popular warrior, man of strict moral principles and wealthy.

When the constellations are strong, then these alone effects which are of course only general, must be foretold in full. If not, these results will have to be modified according to the strength and position of the constellation. A constellation is said to be strong, when a benefic occupies it or aspects it; when it is not aspected by malefics or has their conjunction and when the Moon is generally strong. Take Aswini, suppose at the time of birth, Shani is in it. Moon, of course, will also be there. Moon represents mind and Shani represents sorrow. The combination of these two will be unpleasant and gives evil results. Suppose, on the other hand, Guru or Shukra or well associated Budha is in it, then the constellation becomes strong. If Shani occupies Revati and Kuja occupies Bharani, then Aswini will be between two evil planets and will become powerless to give good results, and as evil influences are close, it might even produce bad results.

❖❖❖

CHAPTER-14
LUNAR INFLUENCES
MOON OR CHANDRA

I shall now give the effects of Chandra or Moon in different signs.

1. **Chandra in Aries**: Round, reddish, handsome eyes, fond of vegetables and hot things, poor eater, irritable, but soon pacified, fond of constant travelling, licentious, weak knees, unsteady wealth, fond of war, caressed by females, clever in serving others, bad nails, head with a scar or sore mark, conceited, eldest of the brothers, good marks in the palm and capricious in approaching watery surfaces.

2. **Chandra in Taurus:** Handsome, majestic gait, big thighs, full face, marks in the face, back or side, liberal, enduring sorrow, brooking no opposition in command, a little hump backed, begetting daughters, phlegmatic forsaken by previous friends and relations, rich, patient, forgiving, happy in middle and old ages.

3. **Chandra in Gemini**: Fond of women, skilful in the art of sexual intercourse, reddish eyes, learned, expert in carrying embassies, ringlets, sharp, witty, clever in judging other's thoughts, good gambler, handsome features, sweet speech, voracious eater, possessing musical faculty, fond of dancing and imperial nose.

4. **Chandra in Cancer**: Fast, but unsteady walker, high buttocks, easily conquered by the fair sex, good friends, astrologer, master of many houses, unsteady fortune, stout neck, short, easily deceived by kind words, obliging and fond of swimming and gardens.

5. **Chandra in Leo:** Irritable, swollen checks, bloated face, yellowish eyes, few issues, hated by women, fond of flesh, forests and mountains, cholic pains, bad teeth or pains there, suffering from hunger and thirst, mental worry, liberal, courageous, steady, proud and respectful mother.

6. **Chandra in Virgo**: Modest, dull, but charming eyes, majestic walk, long broad shoulders and arms, happy, tender skinned, truthful, clever in fine arts. Charitable, learned comprehensive intellect, fond of sexual connection, getting others property, good speech, journeys in foreign countries and many daughters, but few sons

7. **Chandra in Libra**: Pious, regard for elderly or religious men, intelligent man of strict moral principles, submissive to women, tall, prominent nose, lean and shaky body, fond of walking, wealthy, defective organs, skilled in mercantile bargains, getting names, sickly and helper of relations and castemen, but rejected by them.

8. **Chandra in Scorpio**: Broad chest and eyes, fleshy buttocks, thighs and knees neglected by parents and masters, sickly in early life, political respect, yellowish eyes, cruel-hearted, good marks in palms and secret sins.

9. **Chandra in Sagittarius**: Long face, neck and teeth, good patrimony, liberal, poet, strong, clever in speaking, thick neither lip, big ears and nose, hard working, fond of drawing, bad nails, short, but broad shoulders, accomplished, well-read in religion, hater of relations and not won by force, but open to persuasion.

10. **Chandra in Capricorn**: Fond of family, good eyes, collecting money under false pretences of charity, weak waist or not developed, lean buttocks, sharp in understanding things, enjoyable life, lazy, incapable of enduring cold, strong, traveller, miserly, author, fond of low women or hags, destitute of feelings of shame and unkind.

11. **Chandra in Aquarius**: Long and uncouth neck like that of a camel, stiff body with bristle like hairs, swollen veins, long feet, thighs, back and buttocks, broad mouth, stout waist, dear, fond of other's wives, unsteady fortune, doing evil deeds, devoted to friends, fond of flowers, scents, sandal and fine things and capable of enduring fatigue.

12. **Chandra in Pisces:** Enjoying others wealth, gains from pearls and gems, fond of wife and good clothes, handsome, well formed and attractive body, imperial nose, large head, despiser of enemies, easy conquest over them, submissive to women, charming eyes, finder of hidden treasures, learned, good reputation and happy life.

Here, we have to take three points into consideration, viz., strength of Chandra, the power of the lord of the house, where Chandra is placed, and the strength of the sign itself. If all these are strong, the person will surely have all the characteristics delineated here, in a marked degree, but, when they are not so, traces of them will be found. If they are partly strong, some of the qualities will be found prominent, while others will be absent. The readers should take very great care in ascribing these results for their presence or absence largely depends upon sources of strength of Chandra and the house he is in and the lord of that house.

CHAPTER - 15

INFLUENCES OF THE OTHER PLANETS IN THE SIGNS

SUN OR RAVI

1. **Ravi in Aries**: Famous, learned, traveller, earning livelihood by carrying arms and using them, not wealthy; if Ravi is within 10 degrees of Aries, he will be wealthy, commander of many troops, famous.
2. **Ravi in Taurus**: Clever, cloth merchant, dealer in miscellaneous articles and scents, hater of women and fond of music.
3. **Ravi in Gemini**: Grammarian, astronomer, wealthy and polite.
4. **Ravi in Cancer**: Cruel, poor, doing others work, but neglecting his own, constant fatigue by travelling and sorrowful.
5. **Ravi in Leo**: Fond of living in forests, hills, mountains and grazing grounds, stubborn, strong and hunter.
6. **Ravi in Virgo**: Good writer, drawer, painter, poet and mathematician, clever in religious lore and effeminate body.
7. **Ravi in Libra**: Manufacturer of liquors, drunkard, traveller, worker in gold ornaments and base.
8. **Ravi in Scorpio**: Adventurous, cruel, reckless, earning money by poisoning and drugging, losses of property in thefts, clever in the use of weapons and executioner or following some killing profession.
9. **Ravi in Sagittarius**: Respected by well-informed and pious men, wealthy, short-tempered, professor in medicine and carpenter.
10. **Ravi in Capricorn**: Mean-minded, stubborn, dealing in prohibited wears, not rich, miserly and enjoying at others' cost.

11. **Ravi in Aquarius**: Ungentlemanly, poor and rejected by children and family.

12. **Ravi in Pisces**: Pearl merchant or gains from them, and courted by women.

MARS OR KUJA

1. **Kuja in Aries and Scorpio**: Kingly respect, traveller, commander of troops, skilled in mercantile speculations, wealthy, possesses many marks of wounds or cuts, suffers from thieves and fond of womanly pleasures.

2. **Kuja in Taurus and Libra**: Submissive to women, dishonest with friends and relations, fond of others' wives, friendship with quacks, cheats, pendants, timid men and friendless.

3. **Kuja in Gemini and Virgo**: Unrivalled many issues, friendless, grateful, fond of war and music, misery, undaunted and mendicant.

4. **Kuja in Cancer**: Wealthy, gains from sailing on the sea and trading in ships and boats, intelligent, defective in bodily organs and cruel-hearted.

5. **Kuja in Leo**: Poor, enduring fatigue and misery, wandering in the midst of forests and few issues.

6. **Kuja in Sagittarius and Pisces**: Many enemies, minister to a king or chief, famous, fearless and few children.

7. **Kuja in Aquarius**: Always melancholy, poor, wanderer, liar and cruel.

8. **Kuja in Capricorn**: Very wealthy, many children, king or chief, popular, friendly, great personal respect and intelligent.

MERCURY OR BUDHA

1. **Budha in Aries and Scorpio**: Gambler, swindler, drunkard, liar, double-hearted, atheistic, bad wife, robber.

2. **Budha in Taurus and Libra**: Preacher, many wives and children, fond of acquiring wealth, liberal and obedient to parental and spiritual authorities.

3. **Budha in Gemini**: Fond of gups, clever in grammar, logic, music, dancing and drumming, sweet tongue, seeker of pleasures.
4. **Budha in Cancer**: Wealthy by speculations in or on water and hater of his own men and relations.
5. **Budha in Leo**: Rejected by the fair sex, destitute of children, family and wealth, stubborn and traveller.
6. **Budha in Virgo**: Liberal, educated, courageous, intelligent, agreeable, happy, patient, possessed of considerable tact and cunning and undaunted.
7. **Budha in Capricorn and Aquarius**: Poor, clever in mechanical arts, borrower.
8. **Budha in Sagittarius**: Rejected by kings, learned and polite.
9. **Budha in Pisces**: Servile and pleasing, fond of manufacturing shoes or other mean articles.

JUPITER OR GURU

1. **Guru in Aries and Scorpio**: Commander of troops, many wives, children, much wealth, good and loyal servants, forgiving disposition, handsome, loving wife and famous.
2. **Guru in Taurus and Libra**: Sound, healthy, happy, blessed with children, friends and wealth, liberal and popular.
3. **Guru in Gemini and Virgo**: Devoted servants, friends, relations and children, good councilor, often consulted by kings and big men, able to manage complicated affairs with ease and happy.
4. **Guru in Cancer**: Children, wealth, gems, wife, enjoyment of all descriptions, intelligent, educated and famous.
5. **Guru in Leo**: Important commander, good wife, children, happiness, skilful and educated.
6. **Guru in Sagittarius and Pisces**: Ruler of a province, minister or a commander and wealthy.
7. **Guru in Aquarius**: Wealthy, children, intelligent, educated, enjoyment, respect among friends and countrymen, gems and servants.

8. **Guru in Capricorn**: Miserable, poor, fond of irreligious works and hated by sectarian members.

VENUS OR SHUKRA

1. **Shukra in Aries and Scorpio**: Fond of others' wives, spending large sums for them and being frequently cheated by them, incurring religious hatred.
2. **Shukra in Taurus and Libra**: Self-acquired money, self-reliant, commanding the respect of castemen, famous and bold.
3. **Shukra in Gemini**: Knack to please rulers, wealthy, fond of music and intelligent.
4. **Shukra in Virgo**: Mean and unscrupulous, unfortunate wives and careless of reputation.
5. **Shukra in Capricorn and Aquarius:** Popular, respected, submissive to women and connection with women of evil repute.
6. **Shukra in Cancer**: Two wives, beggar, timid, very passionate and melancholy.
7. **Shukra in Leo**: Acquisition of wealth through bad women, good wife and very few children.
8. **Shukra in Sagittarius:** Respected for his admirable qualities, wealthy and intelligent.
9. **Shukra in Pisces**: Wealthy, learned, respected, adviser of kings and nobles and fortunate in all his undertakings.

SATURN OR SHANI

1. **Shani in Aries**: Stubborn, dissembler and neglected by friends.
2. **Shani in Scorpio**: Imprisonment, well thrashed, cruel-hearted, fickle-minded and base.
3. **Shani in Gemini and Virgo**: Miserable, shameless, poor, issueless, bad painter, leader of persons, leader of a band of desperadoes and principal man of his family.

4. **Shani in Taurus**: Incestuous intercourse, many wives and moderate wealth.
5. **Shani in Libra**: Famous, leader of men in towns, influential citizen, commander of armies, wealthy and respected by all classes.
6. **Shani in Cancer**: Beggar, soon losing teeth, motherless, issueless and stubborn.
7. **Shani in Leo**: Ignorant and stubborn, issueless, unhappy and fond of doing others' works.
8. **Shani in Sagittarius and Pisces**: Good death, happy in the end, steward in a king's or lord's house, good wife and children, leader of a town, commander of any army and wealthy.
9. **Shani in Capricorn and Aquarius**: Fond of others' wealth and wives, short-sighted, leader of society, influential citizen, dirty habits, enjoyable life, generous, steady, fortunate and wealthy.

All these results have to be foretold, only when the planets occupy favourable divisions or are strong; if they are weak or debilitated, they leave only traces of the above qualities.

❖❖❖

CHAPTER - 16

RESULTS OF PLANETARY ASPECTS

1. **Birth sign is Aries, or Chandra is there:** If aspected by Kuja, the person will be a leader; by Budha, learned; by Guru, a great statesman; by Shukra, good man; by Shani, thief; by Ravi, poor.
2. **Taurus is birth, or Chandra is there:** If aspected by Kuja, the person will be poor; by Budha, a thief; by Guru, greatly respected; by Shukra, a ruler; by Shani, wealthy; by Ravi, a menial.
3. **Gemini is birth, or Chandra is there:** If seen by Kuja, dealer in arms of all kinds; by Budha, king; by Guru, educated; by Shukra, adventurous; by Shani, weaver; by Ravi, poor.
4. **Cancer is birth, or Chandra is there:** If aspected by Kuja, the person will be fond of waging war; by Chandra, poet; by Guru, professor; by Shukra, king; by Shani, earning bread by the use of arms; by Ravi, bad sight or sore eyes.
5. **Leo is birth, or Chandra is there:** If aspected by Kuja, the person will be king; by Budha, astronomer; by Guru, wealthy; by Shukra, a ruler; by Shani, a barber; by Ravi, a chief.
6. **Virgo is birth, or Chandra is there:** If aspected by Budha, the person will be a leader; by Guru, commander of an army; by Shukra, merchant; by Shani, Kuja and Ravi, successful in doing his own work and after defeated by the intrigues of his enemies.
7. **Scorpio is birth, or Chandra is there:** If seen by Budha, father of twins; by Guru, cringing; by Shukra, washerman; by Ravi, defective organs; by Shani, poor; by Kuja, a ruler.
8. **Sagittarius is birth, or Chandra is there:** If seen by Budha, leader of his men; by Guru, a king; by Shukra, protector of many people; by Ravi, Shani or Kuja, stubborn or showy fellow.

9. **Birth is Capricorn or Chandra is there**: If seen by Budha, king of kings; by Guru a king; by Shukra, educated; by Shani, wealthy; by Ravi, poor; by Kuja, a ruler.

10. **Birth is Aquarius or Chandra is there**: If aspected by Budha, a ruler; by Guru, statesman, by Shukra, fond of others' wives; by Shani, Ravi or Kuja, mean and adulterous.

11. **Pisces is birth, or Chandra there**: If aspected by Budha, witty and humorous; by Guru, a King; by Shukra, learned; by Ravi, Shani or Kuja, sinful.

12. When Chandra occupies her hora, and is aspected by planets in Moon's hora, the result will be good; when Chandra is in her hora, aspected by planets in the Sun's hora or vice versa, the results are bad.

13. **Chandra is in the Navamsha of Aries or Scorpio**: If seen by Ravi, ruler; by Kuja, destroyer of animal life; by Budha, athlete; by Guru, a ruler; by Shukra, wealthy; by Shani, quarrelsome.

14. **Chandra is in the Navamsha of Taurus or Libra**: If aspected by Ravi, stubborn; by Kuja, a monger; by Budha, a good poet; by Guru, holy poet; by Shukra, fond of pleasures; by Shani, fond of others' wives.

15. **Chandra is in the Navamsha of Gemini or Virgo**: If seen by Ravi, a wrestler; by Kuja, a thief, by Budha, a poet, by Guru, a minister; by Shukra, professor of music; by Shani, a clever architect.

16. **Chandra is in the Navamsha of Cancer**: If seen by Ravi, slender built; by Kuja, greedy; by Budha, a hermit; by Guru, a minister; by Shukra, a pimp; by Shani, fond of work.

17. **Chandra is in the Navamsha of Leo**: If aspected by Ravi, revengeful; by Kuja, courted by kings; by Budha, finds hidden treasures; by Guru, strict commander; by Shukra, issueless, by Shani, cruel-hearted.

18. **Chandra is in the Navamsha of Pisces or Sagittarius**: If seen by Ravi, strong; by Kuja, a skilful general; by Budha, witty and humorous; by Guru, minister; by Shukra, important; by Shani, charitable.

19. **Chandra is in the Navamsha of Capricorn or Aquarius**: If seen by Ravi If few issues; by Kuja, miserable though rich; by Budha, conceited by Guru, religious; by Shukra, fond of cruel-hearted and bad women; by Shani, revengeful.

In all these cases of aspects—as in conjunctions—the strength of both the planets who aspects and the planet who is aspected must be taken into consideration. Suppose Moon is exalted in Vrishabhamsha and possesses the aspect of Kuja in Scorpio and suppose Moon is in Scorpio and possesses the aspects of Kuja in Taurus, the results must differ.

❖❖❖

CHAPTER - 17

EFFECTS OF EXALTATION

I have given above relative influences of the planets in their several combinations, but I shall here introduce the reader to a simple method which enables him to find the general condition of the horoscope he is consulting.

1. At the time of birth, if 1 planet occupies its own house, the person will be an ordinary member of his community; if 2 are in their houses, he will be an influential member; if 3 planets are in their houses, he will be its leader; if 4 planets are so placed he will be wealthy; if 5 planets are in their houses, he will be very happy; if 6 planets are so placed, he will live in a regal state; and if 7 planets are in their houses, he will be a mighty monarch.

2. If 1 planet is in a friendly house, the person will be a dependant; if 2 planets occupy such houses, he will be largely helped by friends; if 3 planets are so placed, he will be supported by cousins; if 4 planets are so, he will lead his countrymen; if 6 planets are so occupied, he will be the commander of a large army; if 7 planets are so, he will become a powerful king.

3. If 1 planet is exalted and aspected by friendly planets, he becomes a chief or ruler; if an exalted planet is joined by a friendly planet, he will be wealthy and respected; if 1 planet is debilitated or occupies an unfriendly house, he will be poor; if 2 are so, he will be unhappy; if 3 are so, he will be miserable; if 4 are so, he will be sickly; if 5 are so, he will suffer from imprisonment and bondage; if 6 are so, he becomes a murderer or executioner; if 7 planets are so placed, he will be thoroughly immoral, entirely sinful and completely irreligious.

4. If evil planets in odd signs occupy Ravi's hora, the person will be unhappy, wealthy, courageous and famous; if benefics in even signs are in Moon's hora, he will be tender-hearted, popular, charming, happy, educated, well-behaved and generous with sweet speech.

5. If evil planets in even signs occupy Ravi's hora, he will enjoy the results in the former part of Yoga 4 to some extent, if benefics occupy Chandra's hora in odd signs, he will enjoy the results given in the latter part of Yoga 4 to some extent, otherwise he will be poor and neglected.
6. If Chandra is in the following Drekkanams, *viz.*, 2 and 3 of Cancer, 1 and 2 of Scorpio and 3 of Pieces, the person will be very cruel. If Chandra is in 1 and 3 of Aries, 2 and 3 of Gemini, 2 and 3 of Leo, 2 of Virgo and 3 of Sagittarius, he will become a great murderer or one fond of killing always; if Chandra is in 2 of Aries 2 of Taurus, 1 of Cancer, 1 and 2 of Leo, 3 of Scorpio, and 1 of Sagittarius, he will have incestuous intercourse. If Chandra in 2 and 3 of Gemini, 1 of Leo, 2 of Libra and 1 of Aquarius, the man will be a wanderer without purpose.
7. If the Navamsha of birth falls in Aries, the person will be a thief; in Taurus, one that spends all his money for sexual enjoyments; in Gemini, learned; in Cancer, rich; in Leo, ruler; in Virgo, important; in Libra, a warrior; in Scorpio, a carrier of burdens; in Sagittarius, a subordinate; in Capricorn, sinful; in Aquarius, executioner; in Pisces, courageous. In Vargottama Navamshas, the person will be the leader of the above professions or classes of persons.
8. If Kuja is in his Thrimshamsha (30th division of the zodiacal sign), he will be well matched, courageous, liberal, blessed with jewels, adventurous, charming and popular.
9. If Shani is in his Thrimshamsha, the person will be sickly, widower, cruel, fond of others' wives, anxious, dirty, owner of several houses, many servants.
10. If Guru is in his Thrimshamsha, the person will be wealthy, famous, happy, intelligent, popular, respected, healthy, hopeful and fond of enjoyment.

11. If Budha occupies his Thrimshamsha, the person will be intelligent, skilful in music, showy, political, eloquent, architect, and Pandit, adventurous, popular.

12. If Shukra is in his Thrimshamsha, the person will be happy, blessed with many children, good wife, healthy, rich handsome, cruel hearted, extremely fond of women.

13. If Ravi is in his Thrimshamsha of Kuja, he will be a warrior; if Chandra, lazy; if Ravi is in the Thrimshamsha of Shani, double hearted; if Chandra, fond of killing; if Ravi is in the Thrimshamsha of Guru blessed with admirable qualities; if Chandra, rich; if Ravi is in the Thrimshamsha of Budha, happy; if Chandra, intelligent and educated; if Ravi is in the Thrimshamsha of Shukra, handsome; if Chandra, respect among all classes.

14. If all the planets are in their own houses, the person will have a healthy constitution, successful career, long life and dutiful children.

15. If all the planets are in Kendras, he will be famous; learned, skilful and wealthy.

16. If one planet is in exaltation, the person will get rid of his miseries and will be equal to his castemen.

If two planets are in exaltation, he will become a feudatory prince and will command many. If three planets are in exaltation, he will become a king and will possess good servants; health and children. If four planets are exalted, the person will become an emperor and will possess unlimited wealth and influence; when five planets are exalted, the person will become the greatest ruler of the earth, and achieve great and lasting fame.

❖❖❖

CHAPTER - 18
FEMALE HOROSCOPES

Predictions regarding a woman's complexion, stature and nature and grace will have to be made by the position of the Moon and the birth sign. Her family happiness and the nature of her husband will have to be found out by consulting the 7th house.

1. Birth or Chandra in even signs with the aspect of benefics, will give all the time feminine grace which raises the value of a woman as a housewife. If one of them is in even signs, the women will be pleased with ordinary, modesty, if both of them are in odd signs having evil aspects, she will be thoroughly masculine in her behaviour and will be devoid of feminine grace or modesty.
2. If Chandra or birth is in Aries or Scorpio and occupies Thrimshamsha of Kuja, the girl becomes adulterous before marriage, and if evil planets aspect Chandra, she becomes so even before her puberty; if in Thrimshamsha of Shani, menial servant; if in Thrimshamsha of Guru, an excellent wife; if in Thrimshamsha of Shukra; sinful and unchaste.
3. If Chandra of birth is in Taurus or Libra and occupies Thrimshamsha of Kuja, the girl becomes adulterous; if in Thrimshamsha of Budha, well versed in music and fine arts; if in Thrimshamsha of Shani second marriage; if in Thrimshamsha of Guru, good wife; if in Thrimshamsha of Shukra, moral and respectable.
4. If Chandra or birth is in Gemini or Virgo and occupies Thrimshamsha of Kuja, dissembling; in Thrimshamsha of Shani, barren; in Thrimshamsha of Guru, chaste; in Thrimshamsha of Budha, faithful; in Thrimsham of Shukra, licentious.
5. If Chandra or birth is in Cancer and occupies Thrimshamsha of Kuja, adulterous; in Thrimshamsha of

Shani, kills her husband; Thrimshamsha of Guru, good children and respect; in Thrimshamsha of Budha, painter; in Thrimshamsha of Shukra, licentious.

6. If Chandra or birth is in Leo and occupies Thrimshamsha of Kuja, manly and talkative; in Thrimshamsha of Shani, unchaste; in Thrimsham- sham of Guru, good queen; in Thrimshamsha of Budha, masculine; in Thrimshamsha of Shukra, fond of incestuous intercourse.

7. If Chandra or birth is in Sagittarius or Pisces and occupies Thrimshamsha of Kuja, possessed of good qualities, in Thrimshamsha of Shani, wants little sexual intercourse, in Thrimshamsha of Guru, excellent disposition, in Thrimshamsha of Budha, well informed and philosophical, in Thrimshamsha of Shukra, adulterous.

8. If Chandra or birth is in Capricorn or Aquarius and occupies Thrimshamsha of Kuja, slave; in Thrimshamsha of Shani, fond of vulgar fellows; in Thrimshamsha of Guru, faithful, in Thrimshamsha of Budha, adulterous, in Thrimshamsha of Shukra, issueless.

9. If Shukra occupies the Navamsha of Shani or Shani is in the Navamsha of Shukra or both aspect each other, or if Taurus or Libra is birth and its Navamsha is in Aquarius, the women, not satisfied with men, will have recourse to other women, provided with leather male organs, and enjoys females with unnatural apparatus.

10. If 7 from Chandra or birth is not with planets, not powerful and not aspected by benefics, the women will get a worthless husband; if Shani or Budha is in 7, worthy husband; if 7 is a movable sign, the husband will constantly travel; if fixed, the husband stays at home; if common, the husband will be partly travelling and partly at home; if Ravi is in 7, rejected or divorced; if Kuja is in 7 with the aspect of malefics, she becomes a widow early in life; if Shani is in 7 with the aspect of malefics, she will remain unmarried all her life.

11. If malefics occupy 7, the women becomes a widow; if there are benefics, and malefics in 7, she neglects the first and marries a second husband; if a weak planet is in 7 aspected by a benefics, she will herself be neglected by her husband; if Kuja and Shukra mutually occupy each other's Navamshas, she is very adulterous; if Chandra, Shukra and Kuja are in 7, she commits adultery under her husband's consent.

12. If birth is in Capricorn, Aquarius, Aries or Scorpio and is occupied by Chandra and Shukra aspected by malefics, the women and her mother will be adulterous. If 7th Navamsha from the Amsha Lagna is Aries or Scorpio and is aspected by Shani, disease in private organs; if the 7th house and the 7th Navamsha are good, aspected by benefics, healthy private parts, agreeable to her husband and handsome.

13. If 7 from Lagna is Capricorn and Aquarius or the Navamsha falls there, husband will be old and stubborn; if 7 falls in Aries or Scorpio or the 7th Navamsha is there, the husband will be licentious, revengeful and intemperate. If Taurus or Libra is 7 or becomes the 7th Navamsha, the husband will be handsome, rich and agreeable. If Gemini or Virgo is 7 or the 7th Navamsha, husband will be skilful, learned and agreeable; if Cancer is 7 or 7th Navamsha, husband will be tender-hearted and licentious. If 7 is Sagittarius or Pisces or falls as the 7th Navamsha, the husband will be a gentleman, highly respected and moral. If 7 is Leo or becomes the 7th Navamsha, the husband will be tender-hearted and engaged in several works.

14. If Chandra and Shukra are in birth, revengeful and fond of pleasures. If Chandra and Budha are there, handsome, agreeable, cheerful, skilled in fine arts. If Chandra and Guru are there, virtuous, fond of music, skilful and happy. If Budha and Shukra are there, she will be beautiful, beloved and skilled in arts, and if Chandra, Guru and Budha occupy birth, she is happy, chaste, loving, rich and agreeable.

15. If an evil planet is in 8, she becomes a widow. If a good planet occupies 2 while an evil planet is in 8, she dies before her husband.

    When Chandra is in Virgo, Scorpio, Taurus or Leo, she has few children.

16. If Shani is neither exalted nor debilitated Shukra, Chandra, Budha are powerless, and Ravi, Kuja and Guru are powerful and birth falls in odd signs, she becomes imperious, manly, courted by lovers and reckless. If Guru, Shukra, Kuja and Budha are powerful, and birth falls in even signs, she will be famous, learned in many departments of knowledge, religious and God fearing.

There are great differences between men and women, not only in their physical constitution, but also in their mental characteristics and modes of enjoyment in life. The puberty common to all females is a physical phenomenon, for which there is nothing among the males, which could be compared. Pregnancy and delivery, and then the monthly menses are quiet peculiar to the feminine classes. However much women may boast of their equality with men, there are phases in their life when they require the strong arm of men to protect them and keep them from worry and disturbances. The Rajayogas come to the husband when the female herself does not get the situation. In cases where there is Yoga for wealth, she may earn money for herself; her husband may earn for her, or her parents or guardians may bestow wealth upon her. There are some countries where the kind of marriage contemplated by the science does not exist. Among the brute creation, of course, there is no marriage. But in all cases the coupling of man and women exists, and this has to be read by the astrological rules. Sciences must always be adjusted to countries and circumstances and their spirit must be applied and not their letter. The subject is very interesting, instructive and must be carefully studied.

❖❖❖

CHAPTER - 19

DEATH

Nothing can be more useful than to know the time, the manner and the place of death. Fear of death shows a coward's and a thoroughly sinner's heart.

Men have no business to die before they are one hundred years old. There are two kinds of deaths mentioned in the Shastras. The first is *Kalamrityu* which comes after 100 years and which can be prevented by Yoga practice alone. The other kind of death is *Apamrityu* and this attack humanity at different stages of their existence from the state of foetus to the oldest man before he is 100 years. The Mana or measure of these Vedic year comes to 120 years of solar time. Therefore, it is highly essential for every rational and sensible man to know when he is threatened with Apamrityu and what possible remedies should be taken by him for crossing over those critical periods in his life. Similarly, by a foreknowledge of all his future misfortunes, a person can free himself, by timely and suitable remedies and enjoy happiness.

1. If 8 is occupied by Ravi, death ensues by fire; by Chandra, from water; by Kuja, from weapons; by Budha, from fever; by Guru, from complicated chronic complaints; by Shukra, from thirst; by Shani, from starvation. If the planets are powerful, death ensues under favourable circumstances; if they are weak, under distressing circumstances.
2. If 8 is movable sign, death comes in a foreign country; if fixed one, in his own house; if common one, while travelling.
3. If there are no planets in 8, death must be predicted by the complaint brought on by the aspecting planet. If Ravi aspects 8, death comes by bilious disease; if Chandra, phlegmatic or windy disease; if Kuja, by excess of heat; if Budha, by mixture of all; if Guru, by phlegm; if Shukra, by phlegm and wind; if Shani, by flatulence and death comes from disease in that organ which is ascribed to

the Kala Purusha in that zodiacal sign. Thus, if 8 chances to be Aries and is aspected by Ravi, death ensues by giddiness. If 8 is the Cancer and Chandra aspects it, death comes by flatulent and phlegmatic complaints in the heart or organs about it.

4. If Ravi is in 10 and Kuja is in 4, or both of them occupy 10, death ensues by falling from a peak or by striking against a rock. If Shani is in 4, Chandra is in 7 and Kuja is in 10, the man dies by falling into a well.

5. If birth falls in a common sign and Ravi and Chandra occupy it, he dies by drowning,

6. If Chandra is in Capricorn and Shani is in Cancer, death comes by drowning or dropsy. If Chandra is in Aries, or Scorpio, and is between two evil planets, there will be death by fire or weapons. If Chandra is in Virgo between two evil planets, death results from bandages, or fire or fall from high elevations.

7. If two malefics, unaspected by benefics, occupy 5 and 9, death results from confinement or bandages; if Pisces or Cancer is 8, and its third Drekkana is rising at birth, or if Capricorn is 8, and its Drekkana is rising, death ensues by rope fastening.

8. If Pisces is birth with Ravi, Chandra in Virgo with malefics, and Shukra occupies Aries, he will be murdered by his wife in his house, or through her instigation.

9. If Ravi or Kuja is in 4 and Shani is in 10, he will be crucified, or torn to pieces. If all evil planets occupy trines, similar death happens. If Ravi is in 4 and Kuja is in 10, and aspected by weak Chandra, death comes from sharp weapons. If Ravi is in 4 and Kuja in 10, and aspected by Shani, he will be beaten to death by sticks.

10. If weak Chandra is in 8, Kuja in 10, Shani in 1, and Ravi in 4, predict similar death. If weak Chandra is in 10, Kuja in 9, Shani in 1 and Ravi in 5, death by suffocation happens by smoke, burning by fire, or he will be pierced to death by sharp weapons.

11. If Kuja is in 4, Ravi in 7 and Shani in 10, predict death by fire, weapons through the anger of the king. If Shani is in 2, Chandra in 4 and Kuja is in 10, death comes by worms in sores on his body.

12. If Ravi is in 10, and Kuja in 4, death from horsefall; if Kuja is in 7, and Shani; Chandra and Ravi are in 1, death comes on the rack or by other ingenious contrivances. If Kuja is in Libra, Shani in Aries, and Chandra is in Capricorn or Aquarius, death comes by drowning in nightsoil or in a dunghill. If weak Chandra is in 10, Ravi in 7 and Kuja in 4, similar death happens.

13. If weak Chandra is seen by powerful Kuja and Shani occupies 8, incurable venereal disease, or piles, and death comes by surgical operation in the private parts, or by being burnt there or by nasty worms.

14. If Ravi is in 7, Shani in 8, weak Chandra is in 4, he will be eaten by birds. If Ravi is in 1, Kuja in 5, Shani in 8, and Chandra is in 9, death comes by lightning, by falling from the top of rocks; by falling on the walls of a house or by buildings falling on him.

15. If 8 is free and is not aspected by planets, and none of the combinations above noticed are present, then death must be predicted by that disease which is attributed to the lord of the 8th or the lord of the 22nd Drekkana from the birth.

16. The nature of the place where a person dies may be found by referring to the lord of the Navamsha rising at the time of birth. If the Navamsha is Aries, the place of death will be frequented by sheep and goats; if Taurus, by cattle; if Gemini, private residence; if Cancer, watery places; if Leo, forests; if Virgo, watery places; if Libra, shops; if Scorpio, pits; if Sagittarius, places frequented by horses; if Capricorn, watery places; if Aquarius, a house; if Pisces, watery places. The places of death may also be found by reference to the planets. If Ravi, places of worship; if Chandra, watery places or bathrooms; if Kuja, kitchen and fire rooms; if Budha, place of enjoyment or pleasure

rooms; if Guru, cash rooms, if Shukra, bedrooms; if Shani, dirty places.

Find the Navamsha of birth, and see how much of the sign remains at the time. This remaining time will be the period during which the person dying remains unconscious. If the sign is aspected by the lord of the house, the time of senselessness will be double, if good planets aspect it, the time of insensibility will be trebled; if the house is aspected by the lord as well as by benefics, the time will be six fold.

Now I shall give a few hints which would enable the readers to find out whence a man has come and whither he will go after death. Guru is the lord of Devaloka; Chandra and Shukra are the lords of Pitrolokas; Ravi and Kuja are the lords of Thiryaglokas, and Budha and Shani are the lords of Narakalokas.

Find out who is stronger, whether Ravi or Chandra and the lord of the Drekkana occupied by the more powerful of the two will determine the world whence the individual has come. If the planet so found out is exalted, the person was in a high position before he came to this world; if the planet is moderately strong, he was in an ordinary sphere of life; if the planet is weak or debilitated, the person was in a wretched condition. If there are no planets in 6, 7 and 8, determine which of the Drekkanas in 6 and 8 is powerful, and this will indicate the world to which the person goes after death. If there are planets in 6, 7 and 8, he goes to that world which is attributed to the most powerful planet occupying those houses. If Guru is in 6, 8 or any one of the quadrants and is exalted, the person will have Moksha or final bliss. If Pisces is birth, Guru is in good Navamsha and other planets are powerless, there will be final bliss. The Karmasthana or the 10th house should be well occupied, Ketu in the 12th house from Lagna indicates Moksha. Good planets in the 12th house indicate charitable expenditure and hence favourable lokas after death; evil planets show expenditure on immoral actions and hence inferior worlds of Narakalokas.

❖❖❖

CHAPTER - 20

NASHTA JATAKAS OR LOST HOROSCOPES

There are some who have lost their horoscopes, there are others who have burnt their nativities in anger or disappointment and there are still others whose horoscopes have never been written. The following hints will be very useful for such persons. It is desired that those who have lost their horoscopes or who never had any, should go to a competent astrologer, with suitable presents to command his concentration and goodwill without which no good work could be turned out, and ask him to cast a nativity for them.

The astrologer, after taking the presents, recording the time, position, place and direction of the parties, should proceed to calculate the horoscope on the following rules. Take the time, of question and for the planets as well as the Lagna. If the question time falls in the 1st hora, Ravi must be placed in Dakshinayana, if the question time falls in the 1st Drekkana, Guru must be placed in the same sign, if it is in the 2nd Drekkana, Guru will be in 5, and if it falls in the 3rd Drekkana, Guru must be placed in the 9th house of the question time or Lagna. Find out which of the Dwadashamshas is rising at the time of question and fix Guru there.

If the 4th Dwadashamsha is rising, Guru will be in the 4th house; if the 8th Dwadashamsha is rising, Guru will be in the 8th house. The man's age is fixed at 120 years. He completes the whole period of 120 in 10 zodiacal revolutions; ask the person to touch any one of the organs of the body. If he touches feet, ankles or calves, the age will be within 12. If he touches knees or buttocks, the age will be between 12 and 24; if he touches private parts or testicles, 24 and 36; if navel or waist, 36 and 48; if belly, 48 and 60; if chest or breast, 60 and 72; if shoulders or neck, 72 and 84; if lips or upper part of the neck, 84 and 96; if eyes or eyebrows, 66 and 108; if fore head or head, 108 and 120.

If Ravi is in question time, predict Grishma ruthu; if Chandra, Varsha ruthu; if Kuja, Grishma ruthu; if Budha, Sharad ruthu; if Guru, Hemantha ruthu; if Shukra, Vasantha ruthu; if Shani, Sharadruthu. If there are no planets in the sign, then the lord of the rising Drekkana determines the Ruthu.

If a Ruthu comes out in the Ayanam when it does not occur then have reference to the order of the Ruthu and fix a corresponding one, in which it falls. Drekkana determines the Ruthu, and if the question time falls in the next five parts, fix the second month of the Ruthu. Each sign is divided into 1,800 equal divisions called Lipthas and each Drekkana gets 600 Lipthas. As one Drekkana represents 60 days or two months, a month gets 300 Lipthas. 10 Lipthas will be allotted to each day, and this determines the day of the lost horoscope. This process involves a series of mathematical calculations and one who has no knowledge in them, ought not to attempt this solution. A good knowledge in mathematics is an absolute necessity for all horoscopic work, and one who approaches astrology without this would certainly commit inexcusable blunders.

Another method is thus given: Find in what Bhaga (1/30th) is Ravi and fix the lunar day with reference to that. Thus, if Ravi is in the 10th, then the birth time will be Dashami of the bright half of the Lunar month. If the question falls in Aries, Taurus, Gemini, Cancer, Sagittarius or Capricorn, fix the birth time in the day and if it falls in Leo, Virgo, Libra, Scorpio, Aquarius or Pisces, the time of birth will be night. Take the time of question and find out how many Lipthas have been gained over by Ravi by the extent of the day (Ahapramana) and divide the same by the extent of the night, the result indicates the time of birth in the night.

If it was day, multiply the Lipthas passed by Ravi, by the extent of night or Ratripramana and divide the result by the extent of the day, and the time of birth during the day will be known. Some astrologers say that is the time of birth. There are several other methods of calculations to find out lost horoscopes and they involve calculations of a difficult nature and a good deal of familiarity with astrological formulas. It is not possible to bring them easily before the reader for his guidance in an elementary book like this. I have attempted to teach the reader as much of astrology as could be learnt with the least trouble and devotion, and if I have succeeded in many object, I shall consider myself very well repaid for the labour I took in the preparation of this small book.

❖❖❖

CHAPTER - 21

PLANETARY PERIODS OR DASHAS

With the next chapter, I close my work. It is very essential, for the reader, to know the particular influences of the Dashas or periods and their sub-periods or Antardashas. I cannot, within the narrow compass of this little book, solely intended for beginners, go minutely into the question, but shall confine myself to the general principles which every reader of Astrology ought to know in making his predictions.

1. If Ravi is exalted in Moolathrikona, occupies good Navamsha, well aspected, and in favourable sign, in good conjunctions, he gives spices, tiger's and lion's claws, ivory, skins of wild animals, cruel disposition, travelling, friendship among kings and chiefs, wars, wealth from these sources, inclination to do noble work, fame, invincible, courage and resolution to conquer his foes. When Ravi is debilitated, occupies an unfriendly house, or is in bad subdivisions, in conjunction with or aspected by evil planets, he makes the man hate his wife, children, friends, relations, enemies and thus get into constant troubles with them.

   The man also wastes his money on evil purposes, becomes sinful, quarrelsome with his own servants and dependants, diseased in heart, bowel complaints, loss of power, public disgrace, unaccountable fear of danger, rotten heart, loss of father or paternal relations. The Sun represents the soul, and where he is favourable, there will be elevation of the soul, and when he is bad, there will be depression of the soul.

2. If Chandra is exalted, occupies a favourable position or auspicious subdivisions, aspected by or in conjunction with good planets, he gives the person, during his period, much respect, different varieties of sugar, jaggery, sweet things, gains from superior castemen, fine flowers, sweet scents, plenty of milk, ghee, curds, white clothes, good, jolly company, varieties of oilseeds, pearls, rich food and

happiness from wife and children. If Chandra is weak, debilitated, aspected by malefics and occupies an unfavourable house, he gives to the person, quarrels with kinsmen, female children, drowsiness, patience, evil reputation, religious turn of mind, loss of money and misunderstanding among his own followers, and men of power and position who are able to help him, much mental worry caused through maternal relations, temptations to commit suicide, melancholic attacks, much weakness and numberless petty annoyances. The Moon represents the mind and this will be much affected for good or bad.

3. If Kuja is exalted in Moolathrikona, and lord of favourable divisions aspected by benefics, and is powerful, he makes the man successful in military operations, bold, victor, gains from kings, brothers, sisters, enemies, lands and woolen stuffs, famous, undergoing hair's breadth escapes, travels in different countries, good vehicles. But if unfavourable, there will be cuts from weapons, burns, heart diseases, misunderstanding with wife, children, cousins, brothers, sisters, elderly sort of gentlemen, priests, much thirst from fever, biliousness, venereal complaints, licentious inclinations, irreligious or immoral thoughts and quarrels with his well wishers, loss of physical energy, connection with women in menses, military confinement, and losses in brothers and sisters. Kuja represents physical strength and this will be exuberant when he is strong and physical weakness when he is bad.

4. If Budha is powerful, well aspected, exalted, occupies favourable subdivisions, he gives gain from religious committees, gambling, friends, elderly gentlemen, respect among the educated and intelligent men, gains in gold, brass, bellmetal, horses, lands, popularity, happiness, intelligence, wit and humour, cracking jokes, charitable disposition, patience to serve well under the ruling classes. If unfavourable, the following results

happen—quarrels, sorrow, misery, confinement, mental worry, imprisonment, diseases of all descriptions arising from complications, caste neglect, loss through maternal uncles, derangement or lunacy, confusion and sinful temperament. Mercury represents speech. When he is powerful he will give happiness through speech and conversation, but when he is evil, unpleasantness through this source.

5. If Guru is powerful, predict good, intellectual development, respect, reasonable courage, humility, attractive appearance, victory, philanthropic views, skill in diplomacy, good counsel, encouraging principles of justice, knack to please state officers, gains in gold, horses, children, elephants, clothes, friendship, respect among kings of several countries and great regard among religionists. If unfavourable, there will be mental anxiety from verbal contests, ear disease, hatred among the irreligious and rascally people, service under undesirable masters, misunderstandings among good friends, loss from cultivation, thefts by servants, loss of sons, wife and elderly gentlemen, incurring the displeasures of kings or protectors, unjustified blames, mental worry, misery from various sources and quarrels among his own children, especially sons. Guru represents Gnanasukha or divine wisdom. When he is favourable, he will have happiness through cultivation of sublime ideas, but when he is unfavourable, he will pretend to be philanthropic and thus cheat people and court sin.

6. If Shukra is good, predict taste for music, dancing and fine arts, sweet scents, luxurious food, splendid horses and carriages, good drinks, rich clothes, excellent women, much sexual enjoyment, grand furniture, soft beds, cushions, flowers, sandal, betel leaves, high gentlemanly sense, generous disposition, love to friends, relations and family, success in speculations, treasure troves, agricultural gains and wealth from various sources. If Shukra is bad, there will be hatred of people,

displeasure of kings, quarrels with executioners and huntsmen, foresters and villainous people, grief through friends, loss of daughters, loss of wife or troubles from such sources, rottenness in sexual organs, general weakness, enjoyment with mean women and quarrels with them, losses in silver, clothes and pearls, death of horses, cattle and destruction to carriages, falls and accidents.

Shukra represents sensual pleasures and where he is favourable, he will get pleasures from their enjoyment, but if he is unfavourable he gets misery through these sources.

7. If Shani is good, gains from mules buffaloes, kites, eagles or such other beasts and birds, connection with elderly women, leadership in his community, respect as a citizen, authority over many working classes, gains from inferior grins, loss of father or elderly relations, distrust of the rulers. If Shani is bad, sorrows, phlegmatic diseases, bilious, giddiness, deep-rooted enmity, lazy, dirty, always given to drink and sleep, quarrels with menials, wife and children, injury to limbs, or loss of them by disease or cuts, loss of cattle and lands, evil reputation, dirty houses, unheard of miseries from various sources.

   Shani represents sorrow. He is a very clever planet in giving misery when he is evil, but when he is favourably situated, he minimises the sorrow and increases happiness.

8. If Rahu is good, great power, much courage, success with several classes of influential friends, gains from cereals of all descriptions, good children, wife, servants, travelling, adventurous, headache, piles, internal disorders, immoral thoughts and irreligious tendencies. If Rahu is bad, heart disease, fear from enemies, arson, fires and weapons, destruction of friends and relations, losses from thieves, vagabonds, dacoits, thugs and other rogues, royal displeasure, loss of children, wife, parents and grandparents.

9. If Ketu is good, undaunted courage, political success, good education, friends, houses and eminent position, religious discussions, pilgrimage to holy places, meeting of Yogees and Mahatmas, religious discussions, pilgrimage to holy places, and if Ketu is in a good house, there will be Moksha. If Ketu is bad, trouble from relations, cousin, family, thieves, arson, wild beasts, dysentery, gonorrhoea, cutaneous eruptions, imprisonment and losses from trusted relations and friends.

CONCLUSION

I have, treated the subject very generally and I could not help, as any detailed information would simply swell the bulk of the volume beyond reasonable limits. From the very nature of the subject, and the vastness of the terrestrial phenomena it treats of, no single book treating on astrology could ever be exhaustive or complete in itself.

My English translation of 'Sarwartha Chintamani,' with copious notes and illustrations, is the best book I could recommend for all those who wish to know more about astrology in all its details. My English translation of 'Brihat Jataka' with the complete information collected from the valuable commentaries of Bhattotpala and Jataka Chandrika, with notes on all points are works which should invariably be kept in every educated, European or Indian gentleman's library. No astrological or scientific library could be complete without these works; a sublime subject like astrology could, never even for a moment, be uninteresting or uninstructive, even to casual readers, and if it was neglected by the majority, they simply did so because no author of any merit took the trouble of introducing the subject in an inviting and interesting form in the English garb.

I have led the reader through a great deal of information, which has been carefully and laboriously collected from the best ancient Sanskrit astrological works. I have dwelt on much that invites great reflection and speculation and which might be explained by the thoughtful study of evidence already obtained from various scientific sources, but there is much more, which cannot be so explained and which perchance, may continue for many years quite perplexing to the readers of astrology. I have dealt with a subject, which is full of practical interest and use, but whose true significance and real grandeur, as well as its vast difficulties are, but now beginning to be rightly felt and understood by the educated gentlemen.

The wonderful skill of the ancient Maharishis who found out the results of the planetary influences on the terrestrial phenomena and recorded them in so many formulas for the guidance and benefit of mankind, is unsurpassed by any modern discovery or invention and before we make up our minds to call them fools or reject their works, we must make every honest effort to see that worthy appellation may not be fastened on us by our future generations. Knowledge is power, and must continue to be so, in spite of the clatter of idle mouths, who consider it a fashion to laugh at things which they do not understand and which they do not have the mental capacity to understand. Truth must win and will win the day in the long run. The 'I' of the sceptical man is his bane and makes his mind stagnant and fetish.

VALUABLE INSTRUCTIONS TO THE STUDENTS OF ASTROLOGY

1. Read the first chapter often and often until you remember all the technicalities mentioned therein.
2. Kendras, Trikonas, Panaparas and Planetary Combinations are generally to be taken from the Lagna or birth, unless from the context you are otherwise advised.
3. The ownership of the planets is a constant factor. It does not change
4. Aspects are nearly as powerful as the planetary conjunctions.
5. If there are two or three debilitated planets in a horoscope, the person will have many misfortunes.
6. Do not include Rahu and Ketu, whenever the term 'all the planets' occurs in the book, unless they are included expressly.
7. Good and evil planets give their results mostly in their Dasha and Bhuktis or periods and sub-periods.
8. Never venture predictions on longevity without careful consultations.
9. Combinations from the Moon are as valuable as those from the Lagna and predictions may be safely ventured on such.
10. Conjunctions of evil planets produce bad health, unless they are aspected by benefics.
11. Permanent friendships, etc., of the planets are modified by the temporary relations.
12. If you divide a Rashi equally into two, each is called a hora. If 3 equal divisions are made, it is a Drekkana. If 9 equal parts are made, it is a Navamsha. If 12 parts, a Dwadashamsha. If 30 divisions, a Thrimshamsha. If 60 parts a Shashtiamsha.
13. Acquire facility to fix Lagna correctly, without this you will never be successful in Astrology.

14. Consult the Balarishta combinations in a child's horoscope before you fix the term of life.
15. The sins of the parents will be visited on their children and in predicting the child's term of life, bear this also in mind.
16. Don't draw any inference before you have mastered the whole book and digested its principles.
17. The apparent inconsistencies and contradictions will disappear on a closer study of the several principles.
18. Remember always to fix the positions of the planets yourself with reference to the approved Panchangas or Ephemeris, never venture predictions on kundalies supplied to you by others.
19. Study one system carefully and the others will be easy for you afterwards.
20. Never think too much of yourself. If you do so, you will not progress in any science.
21. The Maharishis of India were no ordinary men. They have anticipated all our doubts and difficulties. The greater the attention you pay to their works, the greater will be your admiration for their genius.
22. Grand things were never achieved by a few days work.
23. Consult first your own horoscope and those of others whom you know thoroughly well and try to justify their character and position in life by true light of astrological principles you have studied.
24. Bring sincerity and concentration into your astrological studies and you will be successful.

CRITICAL PERIODS AND SHANTHIS OR PREVENTIVE MEASURES

Generally, the lords of the 2nd, 3rd, 7th and 8th signs from Lagna are the planets that could inflict death; of these planets, he who is very badly situated will inflict death. To arrive at the conclusion as to the particular planet that would inflict death is a very difficult task. The opinion in this important matter should be given after very careful and mature consideration. Unless the reader makes a thorough study of Astrology, he should not venture to predict this particular point. For the purpose of this synopsis, it may be said that dangers will happen during the 'Dasha' periods of these planets, particularly, in the 'Antar Bhuktis' of planets that occupy the 2nd and 7th houses from Lagna or from the sign occupied by the 'Dasha Natha' or the lord of the major period.

The preventive measures or 'Santhis' prescribed by the great sage Vridha Parasara, if adopted during the currency of such periods and sub-periods, would avoid dangers, the 'Japas', 'Homas' and 'Danas' prescribed by him for the prevention of dangers have been enumerated below:

Sun's Dasha	Swarna Padma Dana (Dana of a golden Lotus flower)
Sun's Dasha, Sun's Bhukti	Suryaprarthana, Rudrabhisheka, Rakta Dhenu Dana (Dana of a red cow)
Sun's Dasha, Moon's Bhukti	Durga japa, Sweta Dhenu Dana (Dana of a white cow)
Sun's Dasha, Mars' Bhukti	Subramanya japa
Sun's Dasha, Rahu's Bhukti	Durga japa and Chaga Dana (Dana of a lamb)
Sun's Dasha, Jupiter's Bhukti	Rudra Japa
Sun's Dasha, Saturn's Bhukti	Mrutyunjaya japa
Sun's Dasha, Mercury's Bhukti	Vishnu Sahasranama japa
Sun's Dasha, Ketu's Bhukti	Suryopasana - worship of Sun
Sun's Dasha, Venus' Bhukti	Lakshmi Sahasranama

Moon's Dasha	Rajata Padma Dana (Dana of a silver flower), Sweta Dhenu Dana (Dana of a white cow) Mrutyunjaya japa
Moon's Dasha, Moon's Bhukti	Do
Moon's Dasha, Mars' Bhukti	Subramanya pooja and Surya Prarthana.
Moon's Dasha, Rahu's Bhukti	Mrutyunjaya japa and Chaga Dana (Dana of a lamb)
Moon's Dasha, Jupiter's Bhukti	Durga japa, Lakshmi japa, and Shiva pooja
Moon's Dasha, Saturn's Bhukti	Vishnu Sahasranama japa Mahishi Dana (Dana of a she-buffalo), Chaga Dana (Dana of a lamb)
Moon's Dasha, Mercury's Bhukti	Lakshmi Narayana japa
Moon's Dasha, Ketu's Bhukti	Chaga Dana (Dana of a lamb)
Moon's Dasha, Venus' Bhukti	Lakshmi pooja, Rudra pooja, Dana of a white cow and she-buffalo
Moon's Dasha, Sun's Bhukti	Durga japa, Durga Dana and Gow Dana (Dana of a cow)
Mars' Dasha	Tamra Padma (Dana of a copper lotus flower)
Mars' Dasha, Mars' Bhukti	Subramanya japa
Mars' Dasha, Rahu's Bhukti	Mrutyunjaya japa, Krishna Gow Danam (Danam of a black cow) and Dana of a she-buffalo
Mars' Dasha, Jupiter's Bhukti	Shiva sahasra nama japa and Dana of gold.
Mars' Dasha, Saturn's Bhukti	Mrutyunjaya japa
Mars' Dasha, Mercury's Bhukti	Suryaprarthana, Vishnu sahasra nama japa, and Dana of a horse.
Mars' Dasha, Ketu's Bhukti	Sri Rudra japa and Dana of a lamb.
Mars' Dasha, Venus' Bhukti	Durga japa and Durga Dana
Mars' Dasha, Sun's Bhukti	Dana of a cow and a gold flower

Mars' Dasha, Moon's Bhukti	Gowri pooja and Durga japa
Rahu's Dasha	Dana of a gold vessel
Rahu's Dasha, Rahu's Bhukti	Naga Dana
Rahu's Dasha, Jupiter's Bhukti	Satha Rudra japa and Dana of gold
Rahu's Dasha, Saturn's Bhukti	Durga japa, Aswatha pooja and Mrutyunjaya japa
Rahu's Dasha, Mercury's Bhukti	Vishnu Sahasra nama japa, Sri Murti Dana (Dana of an image of Vishnu)
Rahu's Dasha, Ketu's Bhukti	Naga pooja and Naga Dana
Rahu's Dasha, Venus' Bhukti	Durga Japa, Lakshmi japa, and Dana of a cow
Rahu's Dasha, Sun's Bhukti	Suryaprarthana, Dana of Til and gold flower.
Rahu's Dasha, Moon's Bhukti	Mrutyunjaya japa
Rahu's Dasha, Mars' Bhukti	Subramanya pooja, Naga Dana
Jupiter's Dasha	Dana of gold
Jupiter's Dasha, Jupiter's Bhukti	Rudra japa, Swarna prathima Dana (Dana of an image in gold)
Jupiter's Dasha, Saturn's Bhukti	Mrutynjaya japa and Chaga Dana (Dana of a lamb)
Jupiter's Dasha, Mercury's Bhukti	Gow Dana (Dana of a Cow)
Jupiter's Dasha, Venus' Bhukti	Dana of an image of Lakshmi-Narayana and a cow.
Jupiter's Dasha, Sun's Bhukti	Suryaprarthana and Dana of a lamb
Jupiter's Dasha, Moons' Bhukti	Dana of a lamb
Jupiter's Dasha, Mars' Bhukti	Dana of gold and lamb
Jupiter's Dasha, Rahu's Bhukti	Tila Homam and Dana of an image of She-buffalo in Silver
Saturn's Dasha	Tila Homam and Dana of an image of She-buffalo in Silver
Saturn's Dasha, Saturn's Bhukti	Mrutyunjaya japa, Tila Dana and Dana of a Black cow
Saturn's Dasha, Mercury's Bhukti	She-buffalo's Dana

Saturn's Dasha, Ketu's Bhukti	Mrutyunjaya japa and Dana of til and gold
Saturn's Dasha, Venus' Bhukti	Dana of a lamb
Saturn's Dasha, Sun's Bhukti	Suryaprarthana and Dana of a gold flower
Saturn's Dasha, Moon's Bhukti	Dana of a white cow
Saturn's Dasha, Mars' Bhukti	She-buffalo's Dana
Saturn's Dasha, Rahu's Bhukti	Subramanya japa and Naga Dana
Saturn's Dasha, Jupiter's Bhukti	Triyambaka japa, of an image in gold
Mercury's Dasha	Dana of a gold vessel
Mercury's Dasha, Mercury's Bhukti	Durga Japa, Vishnu sahasra nama japa, and Dana of an image of Lakshmi Narayana
Mercury's Dasha, Ketu's Bhukti	Dana of a She-buffalo
Mercury's Dasha, Ketu's Bhukti	Durga Japa, Lakshmi japa and Dana of a white cow
Mercury's Dasha, Sun's Bhukti	Suryaprarthana
Mercury's Dasha, Moon's Bhukti	Durga japa and Dana of a Durga image in silver
Mercury's Dasha, Mars' Bhukti	Mrutyunjaya japa and Subramanya japa
Mercury's Dasha, Rahu's Bhukti	Rudra sahasra and Dana of a lamb
Mercury's Dasha, Jupiter's Bhukti	Mrutyunjaya japa, Swarna prathima Dana
Mercury's Dasha, Saturn's Bhukti	Dana of a She-buffalo
Ketu's Dasha	Dana of a Silver vessel
Ketu's Dasha, Ketu's Bhukti	Mrutyunjaya japa and Dana of an image of Umamaheswara (in silver)
Ketu's Dasha, Venus' Bhukti	Durga japa and Durga pooja
Ketu's Dasha, Sun's Bhukti	Siva sahasranama japa and Dana of a white ox
Ketu's Dasha, Moon's Bhukti	Durga japa, Mrutyunjaya japa and Dana of an image of horse (in silver)

Ketu's Dasha, Mars' Bhukti	Durga japa, Subramanya japa and Dana of a vessel filled with oil
Ketu's Dasha, Rahu's Bhukti	Dana of a she-buffalo and Koosmanda Dana
Ketu's Dasha, Jupiter's Bhukti	Rudra japa, Tila Dana
Ketu's, Dasha, Saturn's Bhukti	Mrutyunjaya japa and Dana of an image of Yama
Ketu's Dasha, Mercury's Bhukti	Dana of a lamb
Venus' Dasha	Dana of a silver vessel
Venus' Dasha, Venus' Bhukti	Rudra japa, Dana of a white cow
Venus' Dasha, Sun's Bhukti	Suryaprarthana
Venus' Dasha, Moon's Bhukti	Durga japa and Dana of a deer
Venus' Dasha, Mars' Bhukti	Subramanya pooja
Venus' Dasha, Rahu's Bhukti	Durga japa and Koosmanda Dana
Venus' Dasha, Jupiter's Bhukti	Shiva sahasranama japa, Tila Homam
Venus' Dasha, Saturn's Bhukti	Mrutyunjaya japa, Dana of a black cow and a she-bufalo
Venus' Dasha, Mercury's Bhukti	Vishnu Sahasra nama japa, Tila Homam
Venus' Dasha, Ketu's Bhukti	Mrutyunjaya japa, Durga japa and Dana of a lamb.

❖❖❖

NAKSHATRA SHANTHIS

Persons falling ill in some of the constellations, suffer much. In some cases the illness continues for a considerable length of time and in some cases there will be danger to life also. To avoid dangers, the great sages have prescribed Nakshatra Shanthis. They are briefly described here. For full details, the reader may refer to 'Sri Tatwa Nidhi', a valuable book composed by H.H. Maharaja, son of late Sri Krishna Rajendra Wadeyar III.

Constellations	Santhis
1. Aswini	Danger for 9 days. Aswini Devata Pooja and Homa
2. Bharani	If in last pada of the constellation, death is likely to happen. If in other padas the danger continues from 2 to 11 days. Yama Devata Pooja and Homa.
3. Krittika	Recovery not certain or danger for 9 days. Agni Devata Pooja and Homa.
4. Rohini	Danger for 7 days. Bramha Devata pooja and Homa.
5. Mrigasira	Danger for one month. Soma Devata pooja and Homa.
6. Arudra	Death is certain or danger for one month. Rudra Devata pooja and Homa.
7. Punarvasu	Danger for 7 days. Aditya Devata pooja and Homa.
8. Pushya	Danger for 7 days. Bruhaspati Devata pooja and Homa.
9. Aslesha	Danger for one month. Sarpa Devata pooja and Homa.
10. Makha	When the week day is Saturday, death is likely, Other wise danger for 20 days. Pitru Devata pooja and Homa.

Constellations	Santees
11. Poorvaphalguni	Danger from 9 days to 2 months. Aryama Devata pooja and Homa.
12. Uttaraphalguni	Danger for 7 days. Bhaga Devata pooja and Homa.
13. Hasta	Danger for 15 days. Savitru Devata pooja and Homa.
14. Chitra	Danger for 11 days. Twashtru Devata pooja and Homa.
15. Swati	Danger for one month. Vayu Devata pooja and Homa.
16. Visakha	Danger for 15 days. Indrani Devata pooja and Homa.
17. Anuradha	Danger for one month, Mitra Devata pooja and Homa
18. Jyeshta	Danger for one month, Indira Devata pooja and Homa
19. Moola	Danger for 9 days, Yatudhana Devata pooja and Homa
20. Poorvashada	Danger for one month. Apo Devata pooja and Homa.
21. Uttarashada	Danger for one month. Viswe Devata pooja and Homa
22. Sravana	Danger for 11 days. Vishnu Devata pooja and Homa
23. Dhanishta	Danger for one month. Vasu Devata pooja and Homa
24. Satabisha	Danger for 11 days. Varuna Devata pooja and Homa
25. Poorvabhadra	Danger for one month. Ajekapathy Devata pooja and Homa.
26. Uttarabhadra	Danger for 7 days. Ahirbudhni Devata pooja and Homa.
27. Revati	Danger for one month. Poosha Devata pooja and Homa.

PHALADESHA KALPATHARU

It gives me great pleasure to add valuable information in respect of professions for the guidance of Astrologers and learners which is not reflected in other books. I have collected this information from an ancient Devanagari book, 'Phaladesha Kalpatharu' authored by Shri. Divakar.

The Principal Favourable Occasions

The benefic planet posited in the different houses in the birth chart, their mutual relations, and influences etc. informs about the good and bad happenings of the life of a native and this fact tells us the truth of the theory of transmigration and the mimansa school of philosophy which attaches importance to action, similarly. They say about the bad results also and the time of their occurances, so the good and bad happenings absolutely depend on the good and bad combinations of planets.

The Ten Millionaire

If the lords of 2nd, the 10th and the 1st house are in a benefic place with one of them in exalted sign, the native born is very rich. He earns crores of rupees and enjoys the happy life.

If the lord of 2nd with the lord of 11th house and Jupiter is in the exalted sign and in quadrant house or the lord of 2nd house is in Navamsha and in exaltation also, the native is a ten millionaire.

The Millionaire

If the lord of 2nd house, having full power associated with the lord of 11th is in quadrant house, the native gets every gratification of the world. He is famous and a millionaire.

If the strong lord of the 2nd house associated with Jupiter, is posited in exalted sign and in the 2nd house or in a quadrant house, he is the owner of silver, gold, and famous among the rich society and a millionaire.

If the lord of the 2nd house is in debility in the birth chart, but exalted in Navamsha, then he is the owner of clothes, ornaments, fame etc. He may also become a millionaire.

The Grammarian

If the strong Jupiter is in quadrant house and the lord of 5th house is also strong, the native becomes famous, a great grammarian and a scholar.

The Poet

If the strong lord of 5th house with the Mercury is in kendra the native is a specialist of kavyas and natyashastra and is a great poet.

The Philosopher

When the lord of the 5th house is strong and is in the kendra or trikona with Jupiter and Saturn, the native becomes a scholar of philosophy. He is a sea of knowledge and famous among pandits.

The Mathematician and the Astronomer

If Mercury and Saturn both are strong in kendra or trikona or if Venus and Saturn have a mutual aspect then the native becomes a great mathematician and a pandit of astronomy.

The Astrologer

If strong Mercury is in kendra and the lord of the 5th house is also in kendra the Jataka becomes a scholar of astrology, then he knows about the movement of time and becomes a great prophet.

The Ayurvedic Scholar

When Jupiter and Sun are in kendra or trikona or if strong mars and Sun are in the same position, the native is a great pandit of minerals and Rasashastra, surgery and the Ayurveda.

The Singer, Musician and Dancer

If Venus and Mercury, with the lord of the 5th house are in kendra and trikona and if the lord of the 5th house has an even aspect only, the native has a very sweet voice and he is perfect in singing, dancing and music etc.

The Scientist

When Saturn, Mars and Jupiter are related to each other or located in the quadrant house and trikona, the native becomes a specialist in physics.

The Painter and Photographer

If Mercury is in the shadvarga in a pure situation, in its exalted house or if the houses of Venus and Saturn are well disposed or if Saturn has an influence on Venus, the native becomes a famous painter and earns a world wide respect.

The Playwright and Actor

If Moon, Mercury and Venus are in shadvarga in a pure situation, posited in the kendra or trikona or these planets have mutual aspect then the native becomes a specialist in stagecraft and by this art he wins the people.

The Engineer

If Mercury and Saturn join or have mutual relation with each other and one of them is in its own exalted sign then the native is clean minded, a great engineer who makes the astonishing buildings.

The Greatman

If the lords of the 4th, the 9th and the 10th houses are with the lord of the 1st house and they have a pure situation in the shadvarga and if they are in kendra or trikona or if these four are strong and have mutual influence, the native is a honourable scholar, a great man and the Head of the State.

The jataka, born in above-noted situation of stars, is a honourable, generous, kind, beneficent, brave like a lion and the Head of the State.

The Minister or the Secretary

When the strong lord of 10th house is in a quadrant with strong Jupiter or the same is with the strong Venus in a quadrant or under its influence, the native becomes a Secretary, or the Chief Secretary. If the situation of planets is best with the said combination, the native becomes a minister.

The Deputy Commissioner

Mars, Jupiter and Sun, having full strength and joining kendra or trikona or having mutual aspect, the native is virtuous, famous and becomes a Deputy Commissioner or a Collector of the District.

The Chief Conservator of the Forest

If the strong lords of 10th, 1st and the 9th houses are in Aries, Taurus and Leo respectively, and in kendra and trikona, the native becomes a chief conservator of the forest.

The Journalist

If the strong Mercury, Jupiter and Mars are having mutual influence or relation, the native becomes a great and famous journalist or editor of a big paper or books.

The Versed in Tantra Science

When Mars and Saturn are in kendra or trikona, the native is well versed in tantra science. And if Saturn, Mars and Jupiter have a mutual aspect, the native is a tantrika.

The Agriculturist and Horticulturist

The strong Mercury, Jupiter, and Venus having a mutual influence or relation of place makes the native, a great Agronomist or Horticulturist.

The Joker and Cartoonist

When in the shadvarga, the pure Mercury with the Venus is in its exaltation and in kendra and trikona, the native certainly becomes a Joker or a Cartoonist.

The Army official

If Mars is strong in its exaltation sign and sits with the Jupiter or under its influence in kendra or trikona, the native defeats the army of enemies, the army men salutes him. He is very courageous and becomes a brave army officer or a commander.

The Lawyer

When the strong Jupiter has an influence on Mercury, Mars, and Sun and Jupiter are in Aries, Gemini, Leo, Libra, Sagittarius or in Aquarius, in kendra or trikona, the native is very talkative, wise and a famous lawyer.

The Judge

When the exalted Jupiter posited in Cancer influences the Mercury, Mars and Sun and if these planets are in a strong position in Aries, Gemini, Leo, Libra, Sagittarius or Aquarius in kendra or trikona and Sun is in Aries, the native is a lawgiver, a Justice or a Chief Justice of the Court.

The Foreign Journey

When Saturn, Moon, Venus are in Cancer, Scorpio, or in Pisces and in kendra and trikona or if they have mutual influence, the native goes on a foreign journey.

The Pilot of an Aeroplane

When the strong Saturn is in its exaltation and in trikona or if 9th and 5th houses happen to be Gemini, Virgo or Aquarius, the native is an aeroplane pilot.

The Ship Pilot, Sailor

When Venus and Saturn in Cancer, Scorpio or Pisces and under the influence of strong Mars are in the kendra or trikona, the native becomes a clever pilot of the ship.

The Salvation

If the strong lords of the 8th house and the 9th house are in their exaltation sign and in kendra and trikona and if any one of them is exalted (Deepta) on own sign or if the 8th house is aspected by benefics and similarly if the lord of the

8th house posited in Navamsha in the exalted sign or if the lord of the 8th house is in the same or if the lord of the 9th house is in its exaltation, the native gets Salvation after death.

THE BAD SITUATIONS OF THE STARS

The Burning of Fire

When Saturn, Mars and Jupiter are in a bad house, the person born in this situation of planets is a vulgar, a loafer, who destroys other's property by putting fire.

The Killing

If benefics are in the 8th house and the strong malefics in kendra and in trikona without benefics, the native is a vulgar, killer and notorious among the bad characters.

The Thief

When the lords of the 2nd and the 8th houses are with a malefic in an evil house, the native becomes a thief. He troubles the people by stealing their money and other precious things. He is a man of ill-mind and bad character.

The Woman Abduction

If weak Venus is with the malefic, but benefic in the shadvarga, posited in evil house without relation with the benefics, the native is immoral and abductor of the women.

When one quarrels with the elders

If the malefics are in kendra and trikona and the weak benefics in evil house, the native always keeps fighting with his parents and preceptors and thus is a great trouble giver.

The said combination have been put before the people according to the time prevailing now. It is felt that society is having a rapid change and due to that new subjects are in demand.

It is, therefore, need of the time that Astrologers should always do research on new combinations of the stars and their influence on the natives.

❖❖❖

ILLUSTRATIVE HOROSCOPES

Leaders in Cultural, Ethical and Spiritual Realms

Swami Vivekananda

Moon (mind) deposited in Virgo owned by Mercury (intellect) in conjunction with Saturn, led the man towards the religious and philosophical. Rahu is in Scorpio and Jupiter in the adjoining house Libra and provided the contact with Moon-Saturn. Jupiter helped the blooming of the flower of renunciation (Moon-Saturn conjunction). Mercury in Cancer gave exchange of places with Saturn-Moon combination in Virgo. This added the power of exaltation to Mercury and conjunction with Moon. This combination developed the intuitive faculties, philosophies, propensities and granted him wisdom.

	MARS	KETU	
	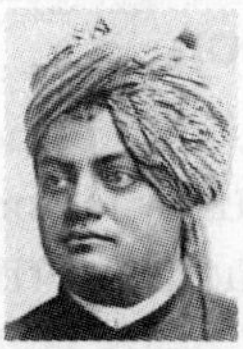		
VENUS SUN MERCURY			
ASC	RAHU	JUP	MOON SATURN

Mars representing ego has in his own house Aries who received the influence of Ketu (which always moves backward) and so developed strength in renunciation. The direct aspect of Jupiter to mars diverted the ego centre valour and heroic effort in the direction of religious propaganda. This book him to the heights of patriot efforts to disseminate the spiritual knowledge of the Motherland.

Moon-Saturn, Ketu-Mars combination turned him into a great Sanyasi (renounced) and endowed him with great wisdom of eternal truth.

Bhagavan Ramana Maharishi

Sun (Atma Karaka) is in conjunction with Rahu and located in Sagittarius and both are opposing Moon-Ketu combination in Gemini. Moon-Ketu combination made the

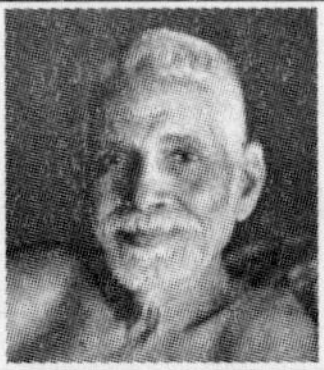

SAT	MARS		KETU MOON
JUP			
RAHU SUN	VENUS MER	–	

native a recluse. Further, Mercury-Venus combination in Scorpio afforded a harmonisation of Atma, mind and intellect. Jupiter is in Aquarius (5th house effects the previous birth) and exchanges places with Saturn in Pisces. This granted the native divine powers (In many Nadi granthas, Pisces is spoken of as the house of God).

Note: Mars is in Mesha (Aries), the house adjoining that occupied by Saturn. This involved the native in mistakes, but the exchange of place with Jupiter saved him and he attained realization. Jupiter's aspect to Mars subordinated the ego to help him grow into a Maharishi.

Talent in Music, Art and Drama

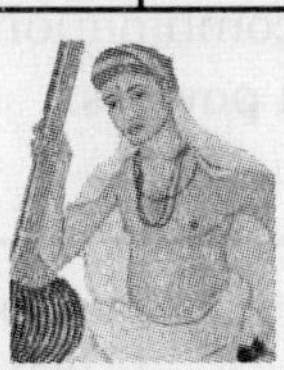

	SUN MER	VEN SAT	MARS
			– KETU MOON
RAHU			JUP

Thyagaraja

The poet mystic: Moon, the lord of the sign Cancer, is in conjunction with Ketu, the divine significator. Jupiter is in Leo, the adjoining house and so his knowledge flowered into wisdom. Sun, Mercury in Aries and Mars in Gemini gave the exchange effect to Mercury and Mars. Venus is in his own house. Taurus and so the subtle influence of Mercury in the house adjoining that occupied by Venus gave the mystic the poetic gift of a very high order with superb musical adaptation of the compositions. It is said in Vedas 'KANTHE RUDRASAMASRITHA HA'. Saturn's presence in conjunction with Venus developed the musical talents of philosophical nature.

The position of Sun in Aries with Mercury and Mercury's exchange of place with mars increased the fiery element and gave him the qualities of heroic natural and slight anger. Venus in the adjoining house down these qualities.

World Famous Musician

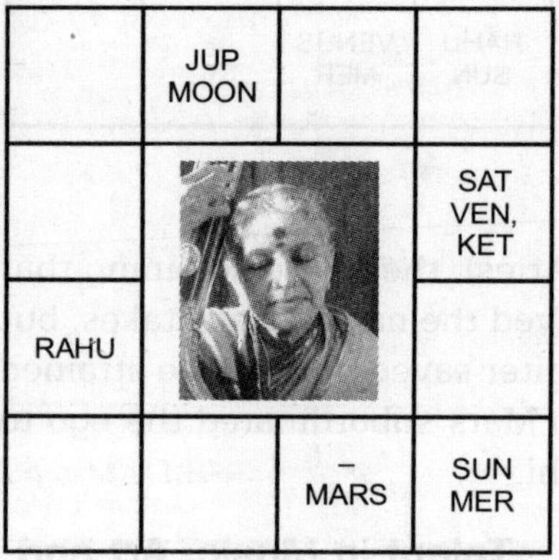

M.S. Subbulakshmi

The Saturn - Venus combination noted in Thyagaraja's chart is also found here. The union of Ketu with the above planets gave here a sweet voice. This triple combination in Moon's house in Cancer gave her artistic and musical talents.

The union of Moon and Jupiter in Aries aspected by Mars in Libra gave her a touch of indomitable nature, but was drowned under the great satwic influence of Jupiter by flooding the mind with divine qualities. This is strengthened by Mercury. Such combinations in Virgo has endowed her with great intellectual powers.

A Great Cine Actor

N.T. Rama Rao

Moon (mind), Jupiter (life) combination in Libra, the rising sign opposed by Venus in Aries show a person with intuitive faculties and dramatic talents, with a pure mind.

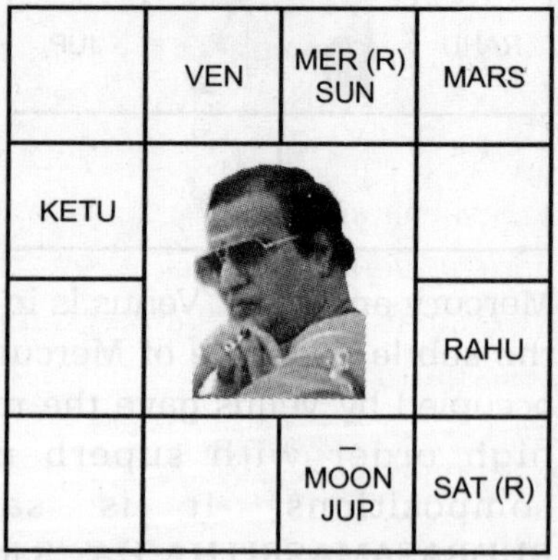

The next factor is Mercury retrograde in Taurus gives sparkling talent and great intellect. Mercury retrograde get (PARIVARTANA) exchange with Mars in Gemini and so Mars get subtle aspect of Jupiter. This endows the man with the capacity to exhibit things known to him without any sense of fear.

Vivekananda, M.S. Subbulakshmi and N.T. Rama Rao have Jupiter-Mars opposition and thus they exhibit the life splendour manifest in them. This brought them great fame. Whether one like them or not they have to admit the great qualities of wisdom, music and dramatic talent respectively manifested in the above three personalities.

Leaders in Religion

Jagadguru Adi Shankaracharya

Atma karaka Sun, Mercury and Venus are in Aries. This endowed the Acharya with a sparkling intellect and he defeated every one in the field of argument. Mars is in Pisces (a watery and God sign) and Jupiter is in Aquarius influencing Mars and made it possible for the Acharya to become the head of a religious institution. Moon is in Gemini opposed by Saturn in Sagittarius. So the Acharya's mind was filled with Ishwaramsa and he wrote the most famous commentaries for the Vedas (Upanishads and Brahma Sutras). Moon-Saturn combination always endows men with wisdom and philosophy in a natural war.

MARS	VEN MER SUN	RAHU	MOON
JUP	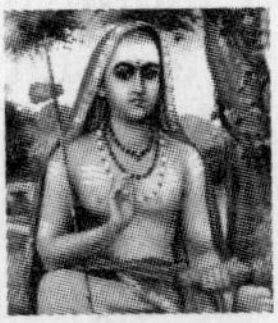		–
SAT	KET		

Jesus Christ – The Founder of Christianity

SAT MOON JUP		KET	
MARS	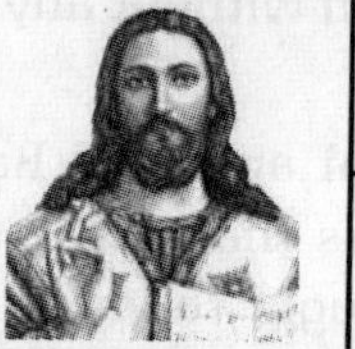		
SUN MERC	RAHU VENUS		–

Pisces is said to be God's house. Its Lord Jupiter is situated in that very house in the case of Pisces. Saturn representing Ishwaramsa is in conjunction with Moon who represents Parvatamsa and both are in Pisces-Jupiter and may be considered to have Saivamsa. As said before, the combination of Jupiter-Saturn, Jupiter-Saturn-Moon always indicate great leaders in religion and philosophy and those who establish religious centres. Christ has this combination in the best house Pisces and Mercury is in conjunction. Sun is in Sagittarius and there is Venus in the adjoining house, but the presence of Rahu in the same house as Venus made Christ not a great intellect. But he did his duty, propagated moral precepts and intuitive faculties were developed as a result of Saturn- Moon combination.

In the propagation of his teachings, Christ had great difficulties and several enemies. This is clear from the position of Mars in the adjoining house to the position of Saturn. Saturn represents past Karma Phala (result) and Mars is the significator of ego. Mars-Saturn combination, opposition or situation in adjacent house always leads to opposition and inimical activities in one's life.

Gowthama Buddha

Aries is in the centre where Saturn and Jupiter are deposited in conjunction with Sun in exaltation and Mars, owner of the house. This special combination made Buddha a great renouncer and one with a firm decision. Jupiter-Mars conjunction made the ego centre to develop highly divine qualities. His undaunting nature mellowed and reached the

	JUP, SUN, VEN, SAT, MARS	MERC	RAHU
			–
KETU		MOON	

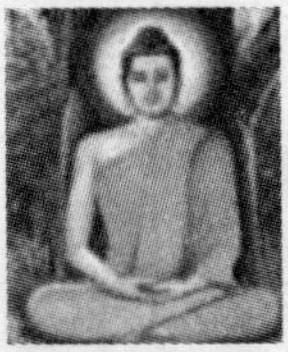

heights of Satwa. Saturn is in debilitation. Further to this the opposition of Sun and Moon had the predetermined harmony of Soul and Atma (Sun) and so Buddha spread his message of Ahimsa. Sun, Jupiter and Mars are friendly planets. The presence of Venus in Aries shows worldly pleasures, but Sun-Mars combination wiped out his kindly position and made him the world teacher. Saturn-Mars combination ignited the inherent qualities of divine knowledge and universal vision and brought about great harmony having gone through the fire of sorrow.

Guru Nanak – The Founder of Sikh religion

		MOON SAT	KET
			–
RAHU	MAR MER SUN	VEN	JUP

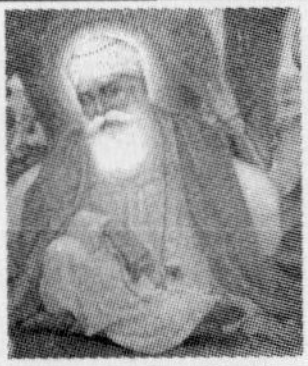

This great soul has Moon in exaltation in Taurus in conjunction with Saturn, while Ketu is in the adjoining house. Gemini owned by Mercury-Ketu's motion is naturally retrograded and so he influences both Saturn and Chandra and granted the native, great renunciation and attainment of knowledge and Saturn made him a religious preacher.

Guru Nanak and Jesus Christ have both Saturn-Moon conjunction. Vidyaranya had Moon in the II house to Saturn. Saturn is of Tamoguna (darkness). Moon represents Satwaguna (Purity and Light). The combination of these two drives away the darkness and spread light.

Shivaji, the Great

MERC	VEN		MARS RAHU
SUN JUP			
			–
KET		SAT	MOON

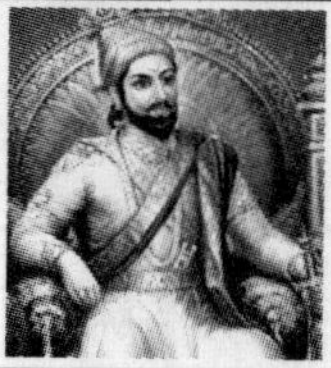

Jivatma planets (Jupiter and Sun) are deposited in Aquarius and influences Mercury in the next house. Shivaji was guided by God all through his life, filled his mind with great love of his country and ruled the territory in a highly judicious manner. Mercury has Venus in the next house, Venus is directly aspected by Saturn in exaltation, Mercury directly aspecting Moon in Virgo, gave Shivaji abiding steadfastness and intuitional flashes. Further Mars representing ego is in conjunction with Rahu made him valourous, undaunted and a man of dynamic action.